Organic Milk Myth

Why organic & UHT milk are much worse for health than regular milk

Russell Eaton

Foreword by Dr. Justine Butler

Published by
DeliveredOnline.com
2008

Title   Organic Milk Myth

Subtitle   *Why organic & UHT milk are much worse for health than regular milk*

Author   Russell Eaton

Published by   Deliveredonline.com
Wokingham, United Kingdom

Email   mailto@deliveredonline.com

Copyright   © 2008 Russell Eaton

Edition   April 2008

ISBN   978-1-903339-24-4

Contents

Foreword by
Dr. Justine Butler

(Senior Health Campaigner at the Vegetarian and Vegan Foundation)

The endeavours by farmers and the food industry to produce organic food free from harmful chemicals are to be applauded. In today's modern world many foods are inevitably contaminated with harmful additives, pesticide residues and other unhealthy compounds.

For decades now the word 'organic' when associated with food conjures up the notion of goodness and well-being. We think, without question, that organic equals healthy. At the very least, if food is labelled organic we generally assume that it is not unhealthier than its non-organic equivalent. This is certainly the case for fruit and vegetables – they even taste better.

However, this is simply not the case for dairy milk. In *'Organic Milk Myth'* the author Russell Eaton explodes the myth that organic dairy milk is healthier than non-organic dairy milk. This excellent book goes even further, showing that organic dairy milk is significantly worse for health in several ways compared to regular pasteurised dairy milk.

The author is not suggesting for a minute that we should switch to non-organic dairy milk. Eaton believes that the best choice is to avoid all kinds of dairy milk and switch to non-dairy milk, a view the Vegetarian and Vegan Foundation (VVF) entirely supports. As senior health campaigner for the VVF, I have researched the health consequences of consuming cow's milk and dairy products extensively. Our ground breaking report *White Lies* reviews a huge body of scientific evidence linking cow's milk and dairy products to a wide range of illnesses and diseases including some of the biggest killers in the West such as heart disease, diabetes, breast cancer and prostate cancer as well as osteoporosis, eczema, asthma, Crohn's disease, colic, constipation and even teenage acne.

Eaton's extraordinary book explains why organic milk, and in particular, all types of UHT (long life) milk could be even worse for your health. In the USA and in many other countries most organic milk is sold as UHT. This book exposes for the first time exactly why UHT milk is so much worse for health compared to non-UHT milk. Whether or not you are a dairy milk consumer, *Organic Milk Myth* is going to surprise, if not shock you.

Organic Milk Myth is a ground breaking book that is destined to have a profound effect on the milk industry, on milk consumers, and even on those who avoid dairy milk. Whether or not you consume dairy milk, this book is a 'must read' for anybody with an interest in their own health and that of their family and friends.

Dr Justine Butler is Senior Health Campaigner at the Vegetarian and Vegan Foundation and author of the highly acclaimed 'White Lies' report. For information about White Lies please go to:
www.vegetarian.org.uk/campaigns/whitelies
Dr Butler holds a PhD in Molecular Biology from the University of Bristol, a BSc in Biochemistry (First Class Honours) from the University of the West of England and a diploma in Nutrition from the College of Nutritional Medicine. She is a regular contributor to national and regional newspapers as well as health and trade journals.

Introduction

Organic dairy milk alone is expected to grow to a $3.5 billion business by 2010, according to J.P. Morgan, the financial services company. Of that, $1.8 billion will come from organic milk sales, double the 2007 level. Organic milk then is a huge and growing business.

In the USA organic dairy products (milk, cream, butter and cheese) accounted for $2.7 billion in 2006. This represents about 4.1 percent of the dairy pie according to the U.S. Organic Trade Association.

It therefore comes as a shock to most people to discover that organic milk is actually more harmful to human health than regular nonorganic milk. How can this be? Isn't organic milk meant to be free of pesticides and be more 'wholesome' whatever that means?

In the context of food, the word 'organic' has almost become synonymous with 'goodness'. At the very least, when a food is described as being organic it is assumed that it is not unhealthier than its nonorganic equivalent.

Generally this holds true: on the whole, organic fruit and vegetables can be regarded as being the same as or healthier than their nonorganic equivalents.

It may seem bizarre, therefore, to suggest that organic milk is actually much worse for health than its nonorganic equivalent. But this will quickly become apparent as you read this book.

About a third of all milk sold in the world today is UHT:

'Fresh milk accounts for an estimated 71.7% of value sales, with UHT products making up the remainder.'[133]

Over 80% of *organic* milk sold in the world today is sold as organic UHT or Long Life milk. The focus of this book is therefore concerned with comparing regular pasteurized milk with two types of milk: *organic* pasteurized milk and **UHT** milk (whether or not organic).

When one examines the latest research in medical journals it becomes increasingly apparent that organic pasteurized milk is not better for health (or even the environment) compared to regular pasteurized milk. And when the research into UHT milk is examined it is clear that UHT milk (whether or not organic) is much worse for health compared to regular pasteurized milk.

This book tells you why this is so, and by simply avoiding organic milk and all types of UHT milk, your health will improve (and you will save money). For the sake of completeness, Appendix C looks at some of the more general aspects of milk.

Sometimes in history hoaxes and myths can become the accepted norm. For example, Kirlian photographers promised to capture on film their subjects' mystical auras, from which could be divined health and emotional well-being. Since its popularization by Russian engineers Semyon and Valentina Kirlian in 1939, New Agers and students of the paranormal have been snookered by the technique's otherworldly coronas of light. Controlled experiments have shown that the Kirlian photos (captured by passing an electric current through the subject, whose "energies" are then recorded on special photographic plates) are the result of moisture and pressure, not spiritual vitality.

History is full of hoaxes and scams, some of which have caused serious harm and distress to people. Organic milk will one day come to be seen as a major hoax, played on society by a multi-billion dollar industry with a vested interest in perpetuating the hoax.

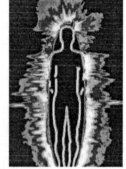

Of course, organic milk is not being compared to Kirlian photography. And clearly, there is no conspiracy. No group of people is deliberately conspiring to create organic milk as a hoax or a scam. Nevertheless, sincere, bona-fide dairy farmers and milk producers are caught up in an industry that is proving to be full of false promises regarding organic milk. This is tragic because, as you will see, organic milk is actually *more harmful* to human health than nonorganic milk, and the truth needs to be told. Prepare yourself for a roller-coaster ride as you read this report and discover the shocking truth about organic milk, one of the biggest hoaxes of our age.

Why organic milk is so unhealthy

In some countries such as Denmark and the United Kingdom most organic milk is sold as *organic pasteurized milk* rather than as *organic UHT milk*.

Some people may therefore be surprised to know that the vast majority of organic milk in the world today is sold as organic UHT milk, i.e. organic Long Life milk.

Look up a definition of 'UHT milk' and it typically goes like this:

> *Ultra-High Temperature processing or (less often) Ultra-Heat Treatment (both abbreviated UHT) is the partial sterilization of dairy milk by heating it to about 141 °C (285 °F), which is the temperature required to kill spores in milk. UHT milk undergoes molecular changes including, in some cases, Maillard Browning depending on the heating process used.*

The growth in UHT milk sales in recent years has been extraordinary. It is estimated that UHT sales will overtake non-UHT sales worldwide by the year 2015.

Why have milk processors embraced UHT milk? Because today's milk is no longer a local product; it is processed in huge processing plants and then shipped to all parts of a country and abroad.

When packaged in aseptic consumer cartons, UHT milk is designed to remain 'stable' at room temperature for up to six months. Its extended shelf life with refrigeration in standard packaging, such as plastic bottles, is up to 50 days – enough time for it to be shipped across a country, or internationally, and sold to customers far from the milk's origin.

In the world today there are two main types of milk, distinguished by the method of pasteurization. These are shown in the following table.

Pasteurization temperatures of milk
(The two main methods)

HTST pasteurizated milk ▶ Regular pasteurized milk, normally requiring refrigeration (organic and nonorganic)	Heated to between 72° - 75°C (161.6° - 167°F) depending on method used
UHT (Long Life) milk ▶ Not meant to require refrigeration until opened, up to 6 months shelf life at ambient temperature (organic and nonorganic)	Heated to between 140.0°C – 150.0°C (284°F - 302°F), depending on UHT method used

The milk industry will often say that UHT milk is the same as pasteurized milk, except that it is pasteurized at a higher temperature. This, of course, is not so because the very high temperatures of UHT (about double that of pasteurization) cause significant molecular changes in the milk.

UHT milk is said to not require refrigeration until opened, and to have a shelf life of up to six months (even nine months in some instances). It has seen large success in much of Europe, where across the continent as a whole 7 out of 10 Europeans drink it regularly.[79] In South America, UHT is growing rapidly, and Brazil is one of the biggest UHT consuming countries in the world. About 1 in 3 sales of milk worldwide is UHT, and UHT sales can be counted in the billions of dollars – It's a big and growing market.

Increasingly, UHT milk is used in an extensive range of products:

• Fresh and recombined liquid milk.
• Concentrated and evaporated milk.
• Dairy creams.
• Flavoured milk drinks.
• Fermented milk products (yoghurt, buttermilk, etc.).
• Whey-based drinks.
• Ice cream mixes.
• Desserts (custards and puddings).
• Protein drinks.
• Baby foods.
• Beverage whiteners for such things as tea and coffee.
• Soups, sauces, purees, and dressings containing dairy products.
• Airline catering.
• Milk for the military.

In some countries virtually all milk consumption is UHT. In France, Belgium and Spain, for example, over 95% of all milk sold is UHT, whereas in the United Kingdom it is about 10%, so there is great variation.

When it comes to organic milk, growth in demand in the USA is increasing at about 25% - 30% per year according to the American USDA. Similar growth in demand for organic milk applies to other parts of the world.

The two biggest reasons for buying organic milk in the USA are the perceptions that it has no hormones and no antibiotics. (Source: NMI Omnibus, 2006).

As we shall see later, these perceptions are misplaced.

As mentioned in the Introduction, over 80 percent of organic milk (worldwide) is sold as UHT. In countries where most milk is UHT, virtually all *organic* milk is UHT. If organic milk is being sold from non-refrigerated shelving you know the milk must be UHT. However, many retailers are choosing to sell some of their organic UHT milk from refrigerated shelving to give the impression that the milk is 'fresh' rather than 'long life'. Always check the carton if you want to avoid UHT milk.

In a poll done by OMSCO (UK Organic Milk Suppliers Cooperative) in June 2006, nearly 1,700 people all over the United Kingdom where questioned about their perception of organic milk.

It was discovered that in the UK about 61 percent of all milk consumers buy organic milk frequently. A similar percentage is likely to apply to other first world countries.

The poll also discovered two other beliefs held by consumers: (i) 91% believed the welfare of organic cows to be either good or excellent, and (ii) the health benefits of organic milk were the most significant factor in deciding to buy organic milk. As we shall see later on, neither of these two assumptions hold true.

In the North American market, consumers have been uneasy about consuming UHT milk which is not delivered under refrigeration, and have been much more reluctant in buying it. But this is changing and UHT sales in the USA are growing fast. Many milk products in North American foods are made using UHT milk, such as McDonalds McFlurries.

Furthermore, virtually all *organic* milk in the USA is UHT.

Even though most organic milk in the world today is UHT, in some of the smaller countries (where milk distribution is on a smaller scale and the climate not so hot) this is not so. For example, in the UK, Denmark and Holland most *organic* milk is pasteurized rather than UHT.

Another reason for the preponderance of UHT as a pasteurizing method for organic milk is the fear of disease. Organic farming methods greatly increase the amount of pathogens that come into contact with so-called organic cows. It is feared by some that mere pasteurization is not enough, and that the higher heat treatment of UHT is required to be safe from pathogens.

Is UHT worse for health than regular pasteurized milk? The answer is yes for a variety of reasons. What follows is a summary of why UHT is worse for health *compared to regular pasteurized milk*. These issues (with supporting evidence) are examined in greater detail throughout this book.

- UHT gives you a greater amount of cancer-causing hormones known as IGF-1. This subject is examined in detail in the next chapter.

- UHT gives you a greater amount of toxins (heavy metals and dioxins).

- UHT gives you a greater amount of damaged proteins, increasing the risk of neurodegenerative diseases such as Alzheimer's, Parkinson's, and Huntington's disease.

- UHT gives you a greater amount of harmful galactose, increasing the risk of cataracts, infertility and cancer.

- UHT spoils more quickly once opened, typically lasting no more than about three days in the fridge. This compares with 5 to 8 days for regular pasteurized milk. The reason for this is that the UHT pasteurization process kills anti-bacterial enzymes that normally would help to keep milk fresh.[84]

- UHT is more acid-forming once consumed compared to regular pasteurized milk. The more acidic a food the worse it is for health.

- UHT causes more respiratory congestion and worse immunity caused by casein.

- UHT is less nutritious because enzymes, minerals and some vitamins are lost during the UHT pasteurization process.

UHT and Cancer

To say that UHT is the worst kind of milk to consume would be an understatement – it is not only unhealthy per se, but may actually increase the risk of cancer and brain disease. This is so for both organic UHT and nonorganic UHT milk.

As you will see, if you must consume dairy milk, any kind of UHT milk (organic or nonorganic) is a bad choice.

One of the worst aspects of UHT milk is the amount of cancer-causing hormones it gives you (significantly more than regular pasteurized milk!).

This is how milk gives you cancer-causing hormones, summarized in the following five points:

1. All kinds of milk whether raw, pasteurized, organic or UHT contain cancer-causing hormones known as IGF-1(*Insulin-like Growth Factor 1*). This IGF-1 is contained inside the tiny globule membranes that hold the milk fat.

2. UHT and regular pasteurized milk contain similar amounts of IGF-1. The difference is that with UHT more of the IGF-1 enters into the bloodstream (the way this happens is explained in the chapter *The Lethal UHT Effect*).

3. IGF-1 is a natural growth hormone that will enable the future calf to grow. All kinds of dairy milk have IGF-1 unless all the fat in milk is removed. IGF-1 from dairy milk is known to increase the risk of cancer in humans (see Appendix B for the evidence).

4. When milk is consumed, the IGF-1 hormone enters the bloodstream and from there it is

deposited in many parts of the body, increasing the risk of cancer.

Why do cows produce harmful IGF-1? Virtually all dairy cows (including 'organic' dairy cows) are kept in a state of almost continuous pregnancy so as to maximize milk production. This continuous state of pregnancy produces milk rich in IGF-1. No amount of organic diligence and no amount of pasteurization gets rid of these harmful bovine IGF-1 hormones – they are a natural component of all dairy milk. Many highly regarded studies show that IGF-1 in milk causes a multitude of diseases in humans.

Some milk producers try to justify their stance (vis-à-vis cancer-causing hormones in milk) by saying that they are not allowed by law to give **growth** hormones to dairy cows. Any such statement would be both disingenuous and misleading. In the United Kingdom, for example, growth hormones are banned on all dairy farms, not just organic farms. In the United States some growth hormones are banned and others are allowed.

But IGF-1 is not something that can be banned – it is produced naturally by the cow's body as a result of pregnancy. So IGF-1 is a natural growth hormone found in all types of milk and it cannot be removed.

'IGF-1 in milk was originally thought to be destroyed by digestion, unable to reach the bloodstream where it could affect cancer rates. Although IGF-1 by itself doesn't survive digestion, studies conducted after 1993 indicate that casein, the main protein in milk, protects most IGF-1 from digestion.'[22]

The harm caused by IGF-1 to human health reads like a horror story. Here are just a few of the many studies showing how IGF-1 in dairy milk (organic or nonorganic) causes illness:

1. *IGF-1 survives pasteurization and human digestion and has been identified as the key factor in breast cancer growth.*[5]

2. *IGF-1 from dairy milk is particularly harmful to humans because it has the same DNA composition as natural human growth hormone, and as a result growth hormones from cow's milk are fully assimilated into the human body. By drinking cow's milk, we deliver IGF-1 right into the body's cells.*[6] Note: IGF-1 causes cancer because *all types* of cancer growth depend on our body's Insulin Growth Factor to take hold and grow. When IGF-1 from dairy milk is consumed it increases the risk of cancer by allowing cancers to grow and proliferate much more vigorously.

3. *Milk, whether human or dairy, is a hormonal delivery system designed to help the progeny grow quickly. Dairy milk is specifically designed for rapid growth of calves. When humans consume a cocktail of hormones designed for calf growth it plays havoc with the human body in many different and harmful ways.*[7]

4. *IGF-1 is critically involved in the aberrant growth of human breast cancer cells.*[8]

5. *We manufacture IGF-1 in our bodies. We also consume IGF-1 in pasteurized, homogenized dairy milk. The tiny homogenized fat globules carry IGF-1 from milk through the stomach and gut into the bloodstream where they can circulate through the body to exert powerful growth effects. This IGF-1 allows cancers to grow.*[9]

6. *Estrogen regulation of IGF-1 in breast cancer cells would support the hypothesis that IGF-1 has a regulatory function in breast cancer.*[10]

7. IGF-1 is a potent growth factor for cellular proliferation in the human breast carcinoma cell line.[11]

8. IGF-1 plays a major role in breast cancer cell growth.[12]

9. IGF-1 produces a 10-fold increase in RNA levels of cancer cells. IGF-1 appears to be a critical component in cellular proliferation.[13]

10. IGF-1 accelerates the growth of breast cancer cells.[14]

11. A strong positive association was observed between IGF-1 levels and prostate cancer risk.[15]

12. IGF-1 can affect the proliferation of breast epithelial cells, and is thought to have a role in breast cancer.[16]

13. IGF-1 strongly stimulates the proliferation of a variety of cancer cells, including those from lung cancer.[17]

14. IGF-1 is widely involved in human carcinogenesis. A significant association between IGF-1 and an increased risk of lung, colon, prostate, and pre-menopausal breast cancer has recently been reported.[18]

15. A raised level of IGF-1 has been associated with breast cancer for women and prostate cancer for men.[19]

16. By continuing to drink milk, one delivers the most powerful growth hormone [IGF-1] in nature to his or her body. That hormone has been called the key factor in the growth of breast, prostate, and lung cancer. At the very best, or worst, this powerful growth hormone instructs all cells to grow. This might be the reason that Americans

are so overweight. At the very worst, this hormone does not discriminate. When it finds an existing cancer, usually controlled by our immune systems, the message it delivers is: GROW![9]

17. *Some dairy milk samples also show noticeable concentration of a growth hormone given to cows to promote their growth and increase milk production. Being fat-soluble, hormones are more concentrated in the cream. Hormones in milk are a serious threat to health because even at very low concentrations, they can cause severe imbalance of our physiologic system. They have also been implicated in many types of cancers and decreased resistance to infections and diseases. Though prohibited in some parts of the world, unscrupulous farmers continue to use hormones. Whatever a cow eats shows up in her udders. Grass, silage, straw, cereals, roots, tubers, legumes, oilseeds, oilcakes, and milk by-products, which contain a variety of chemical additives, make the diet of modern cow. The diet of cows is rife with pesticides, fertilizers, herbicides and traces of heavy metals along with chemicals from spoilage. With each glass of milk shoved down little Jane's or Johnny's throat, comes the increased chance of their developing atherosclerosis, cancer, autoimmune diseases, infections and a host of other diseases still unidentified, when they reach adulthood.*[20]

18. *Several studies show that IGF-1 in organic and nonorganic milk accelerates early puberty in young boys and girls. This makes you more prone to develop cancer later in life. Also, early puberty in girls causes depression, aggressiveness, social withdrawal, moodiness, behavioural problems, and a greater tendency to*

smoke and take drugs. Worse still, early puberty in a girl increases the risk of osteoporosis later in life.[7]

19. *Both laboratory and epidemiological studies have demonstrated that elevated levels of IGF-1 are associated with increases in several types of cancers in humans.*[21]

20. *IGF-I has been identified as a key factor in breast cancer.*[68]

Many other scientific studies suggest IGF-1 in milk survives digestion and enters the bloodstream in sufficient quantities to potentially trigger increased cancer rates. For more information and supporting evidence concerning IGF-1 please see Appendix B.

IGF-1 occurs in all kinds of dairy milk, in all countries, whether raw, pasteurized, organic, nonorganic, homogenized, ultra-pasteurized, or whether made into yogurt, cheese, butter.
If you consume dairy, you consume IGF-1

What about organic UHT?

Does organic milk give you more IGF-1 than regular pasteurized milk? The answer is YES because although the amount of IGF-1 may be similar in both kinds of milk, organic UHT milk will deliver a higher amount of IGF-1 into the body and the bloodstream.

As explained in the chapter *The Lethal UHT Effect*, more IGF-1 gets delivered into the body courtesy of the micronized fat globules created by high intensity homogenization. But regular pasteurized milk is also homogenized so what's the difference?

The difference is that UHT milk contains a higher proportion of smaller fat globules as a consequence of the ultra high homogenization pressure and the ultra high pasteurization temperature.

This helps the fat globules to be digested and absorbed into the body more efficiently (the task of breaking food down to smaller particles is made less onerous for the digestive system).

To clarify further: all types of milk (whether or not organic) contain similar amounts of IGF-1. But UHT milk (both organic and nonorganic) sends more IGF-1 into the body to cause harm.

This is alarming because the bulk of milk consumed in the world today is UHT. And the bulk of organic milk consumed is UHT. In the USA alone, 80% of organic milk is UHT.[25]

The following table shows UHT milk in Europe as a percentage of total consumption. In countries such as Belgium, Spain and France virtually all milk (organic and nonorganic) is UHT – see next page.

UHT milk in some European countries as a percentage of total consumption			
1	96.7 – Belgium	10	35.1 – Hungary
2	95.7 – Spain	11	20.3 – Austria
3	95.5 – France	12	20.2 – Netherlands
4	92.9 – Portugal	13	
5	71.4 – Czech Rep	14	10.9 – Ireland
6	66.1 – Germany	15	5.5 – Sweden
7	49.8 – Italy	16	5.3 – Norway
8	48.6 – Poland	17	2.4 – Finland
9	35.5 – Slovakia	18	0.9 – Greece
			0.0 – Denmark
Source: Euromonitor International			

In countries with high UHT consumption, virtually all *organic* milk is sold as UHT. But even in countries where the percentage of UHT consumption is not particularly high, such as the USA and Canada, the percentage of organic milk sold as UHT is very high.

This is because most organic milk is produced by small dairy farmers and the supply chain from cow to consumer is not so well established. So in large or hot-weather countries such as Spain, France, the USA and Australia, most organic milk tends to be UHT.

It is much more practical to store and distribute organic and nonorganic UHT when there are few or no refrigeration requirements.

In smaller (and colder) countries such as Denmark, Finland, Ireland and the United Kingdom most organic milk is sold as pasteurized rather than as UHT. This is possible because of climatic conditions and the shorter geographical distances in the supply chain.

It is clear that many milk producers are not advertising the fact that they are providing UHT milk; the words 'Ultra Heated', 'UHT' or 'Long Life' are written (if at all) in very small letters on the milk carton, and the milk is typically sold in the refrigerated section even though the milk can be kept unrefrigerated until opened.

Another ruse that has become apparent is that many milk producers package UHT milk in cartons and plastic bottles identical to those containing regular pasteurized milk.

When buying milk from the refrigerated section of a retailer, you should check whether it is pasteurized or UHT as it could be either. And always remember that whatever the country and whatever the type of milk, if it is being sold on shelves that are not refrigerated, the milk has to be UHT!

In the USA, Horizon – the major *organic brand*, is UHT as are virtually all U.S. national brands. In Europe and other parts of the world there is an increasing trend to produce all kinds of milk as UHT. Gradually the proportion of UHT milk is expected to increase compared to non-UHT milk. One reason for this is global warming: there is a worldwide strategy to ensure that some 90 per cent of milk on sale will not require refrigeration by 2020.[71]

This chapter is concluded with a point of clarification for consumers of American milk.

Milk consumers in the United States and some other countries such as Brazil should note that most regular pasteurized milk comes from cows that have been given synthetic growth hormones, known as rBGH or rBST (brand name Posilac). These synthetic growth hormones are given to cows to make them produce more milk than they normally would.

Some studies show that synthetic growth hormones in milk can increase the risk of cancer in human milk consumers. A study of this subject is beyond the scope of this book, and in any event the use of synthetic growth hormones is banned in organic milk.

Consequently, a big selling point for organic milk in the USA and some other countries is that it does not contain synthetic growth hormones. However, this is a mute point since all kinds of dairy milk are rich in growth hormones (known as IGF-1). Clearly, organic milk without synthetic hormones is going to be better than nonorganic milk with synthetic hormones.

But it does not follow that organic milk without synthetic hormones is therefore a healthy product to consume. Whether the milk is organic, nonorganic, UHT, raw, pasteurized, skim or semi-skim, *all types of dairy milk* contain high amounts of IGF-1 bovine hormones that are known to cause cancer (for the evidence see Appendix B).

This is why confusion can arise when it comes to milk labelling in the USA. Some organic milk labelling states that the milk is "hormone free" or "rBST free". This can be misleading because, as stated, *all kinds of dairy milk* contain the harmful IGF-1 growth hormones. Therefore no organic milk should be labelled as "hormone free" or imply that it is free of hormones.

The Horror of Homogenization

All kinds of pasteurized and UHT milk are also homogenized (including organic milk).

Milk straight from the cow contains cream, which rises to the top. Homogenization is a process that breaks up the fat globules and distributes them evenly throughout the milk so that they do not rise. This process greatly increases the surface area of fat exposed to air by four to sixfold.[123]

When it comes to UHT the homogenization process is much more intense, increasing the surface area of fat globules by eight to tenfold.[80] This in turn increases oxidation and the susceptibility to spoilage.

Surface area of fat is increased by homogenization because many smaller fat globules have a bigger *total* surface area than fewer bigger fat globules.

A sharp increase in the fat globules' specific surface area was observed for DSI (140°C heat-treated) milk.[84] Note: 'DSI' refers to a method of pasteurization used for UHT.

If raw milk is homogenized without pasteurization it goes rancid very quickly. Therefore pasteurization is usually carried out first, immediately followed by homogenization. With UHT milk, homogenization is usually carried out first, followed by pasteurization.

For some dairy products homogenization is carried out both before and after pasteurization. Different homogenization temperatures may be used depending on quality of milk, the final product being made, type of equipment, degree of pressure used, and storage/distribution factors.

When milk is homogenized it is forced through tiny holes or tubes at high pressure to break the fat down to very small micronized globules.

Homogenization can cause health problems for the following three specific reasons examined below:

1. **Increase in toxins.**

2. **Increase in harmful body fat.**

3. **Increase in allergy.**

***

1. *Increase in toxins.* The tiny homogenized fat globules that enter the bloodstream act as a 'conveyor-belt' for harmful toxins, hormones, heavy metals, dioxins, IGF-1, etc. that may be present in the milk and *other food* we may be consuming at the time.

Normally, our body is protected from the harmful elements of consumption. Our digestive system and liver act to filter out harmful things in the food we eat. But when dairy milk is consumed, the tiny homogenized fat globules 'absorb' some of these harmful elements making them more likely to be digested and carried into the body (instead of being excreted). This is explained more fully in the chapter *The Lethal UHT Effect.*

This homogenization process, referred to as **micronization of fat**, is so effective that some medications are encapsulated into micronized fat as a way of delivering them into the body orally instead of using needle injections.

Although the amount of toxins and heavy metals we consume in the food we eat may be very small, they accumulate in the body over a period of time. As heavy metals such as cadmium, mercury and lead are highly toxic, only small amounts are needed for serious illness to develop. Dairy milk provides more heavy metals than just about any other kind of food because of their concentrated presence in milk, combined with a highly effective delivery system.

Claims of lower levels of toxins in organic milk vs. conventional milk appear to be unfounded.[1] For example, two European studies indicate higher levels of aflatoxin M1 in organic milk and cheese compared with conventional products.

Aflatoxin M1 is a toxic fungus found in milk or milk products obtained from livestock that have ingested contaminated feed. Ghidini, et al.[32] observed that *'aflatoxin M1 contamination in some, but not all, samples of organic milk (35 ug/l) was significantly higher than those of conventional milk (21 ug/l)'.*

Vallone, et al.[33] research results showed *'the presence of aflatoxin M1 in organic cheese samples occurred frequently, but at low levels (<0.25 mg/kg cheese). This occurrence has been hypothesized to be due to ineffective pesticide treatment of organic grain crops, a not infrequent occurrence'.*

(For more information on toxins in milk please see *'The Organic Milk Toxins Myth'* in this book)

2. *Increase in harmful body fat.* Homogenization has the effect of sending more harmful fat into the body. This harmful fat is not used as energy or as useful nutrition. Instead, it causes illness and heart disease or ends up being stored as surplus body fat. This occurs for four reasons:

i. The homogenized fat globules are made of long chain saturated fatty acids (14, 16 and 18 chain carbon atoms). The 14 and 16 long chain fatty acids are known to increase the level of harmful (oxidized) cholesterol in the bloodstream, leading to arterial disease.

ii.   Saturated animal fat consumed in the diet cannot be used by the body unless it is first converted into non-saturated fat. Since the body cannot easily convert 14 and 16 chain fatty acids into non-saturated fat, they are dumped by the bloodstream, i.e. stored as surplus body fat.

Healthy Artery with Normal Blood Flow

Plaque Deposits Restricting Blood Flow

iii.   The 14 and 16 chain homogenized fatty acids are more harmful than saturated fats (virtually on a par with trans-fatty acids). This is so because, like trans-fatty acids, they enter the body and become lodged within the cell membranes of various organs where they cause harm. They can do this because of their small size and because their molecular composition prevents them from being broken down and used by the body.

iv.   Although the 14 and 16 chain homogenized fatty acids are technically classified as saturated fat they behave more like trans-fatty acids inside the body. In pasteurized whole milk, most of the saturated fat is made up of 14 and 16 chain fatty acids (about 67%). This means that about two thirds of the saturated fat from dairy milk is not only fattening, but harmful on a par with trans-fatty acids.

Look at the label on a carton of pasteurized whole milk (3% milk) in the USA and you will see that it says it contains a zero amount of trans-fatty acids (or It may not mention trans-fatty acids at all). In reality, all milk contains trans-fatty acids, but when the amount is below 0.5% per 100g of milk the authorities allow the labelling to show the amount as zero. This misrepresentation of trans-fats is further compounded by the similarity of the tiny homogenized fat globules to trans-fats, in terms of the harm they do to the body.

3. *Increase in allergy.* We have stated that during homogenization there is a tremendous increase in the surface area of the fat globules (lots of small fat globules have a bigger total surface area than fewer bigger fat globules).

This greater surface area makes the fat globules bind with a much greater portion of casein and whey proteins.[13] This may account for the increased allergenicity of homogenized pasteurized milk.

During digestion, the micronized fat globules with their coating of casein and whey proteins are broken down and absorbed (transferred through the intestinal wall) into the body. Homogenization causes much greater absorption of these super-harmful proteins. Without homogenization, less casein and damaged whey proteins are absorbed because they are less available to the digestive system, i.e. less broken down and 'spread out' over the surface area of fat globules).

The case against homogenized milk is so overwhelming that virtually no health professional (unless allied to the milk industry) can say that it is good for you. Here are some extracts from some of the research:

- *Heart disease is proportional to the amount of homogenized milk consumed in a country.*

Finland has the highest consumption... and the highest heart disease rate followed by the US. Nicholas, Samsidis, MS, *Homogenized - How Homogenized Milk Triggers Heart and Circulatory Disease,* Park City Pr; June 1994.

- *Milk and milk products gave the highest correlation coefficient to heart disease.* Survey of Mortality Rates and Food Consumption Statistics of 24 Countries, Medical Hypothesis, 7:907-918, 1981.

- *Milk consumption correlates positively with ... coronary mortality. In comparisons between 17 countries, there is a good correlation between levels of mortality from heart disease.* European Journal of Clinical Nutrition, 48, 1994.

- *Milk positively related to coronary heart disease for all 40 countries studied.* Circulation, 1993; 88(6).

- *For heart disease milk was found to have the highest statistical association for males aged 35+ and females aged 65+.* Alternative Medical Review, 1998 Aug, 3:4.

- *The fat in commercial milk is homogenized, subjecting it to rancidity. When milk is homogenized, small fat globules surround the xanthine oxidase and it is absorbed intact into your blood stream. There is some very compelling research demonstrating clear associations with this absorbed enzyme and increased risks of heart disease.* Dr. Joseph Mercola (licensed physician).

As stated, virtually all commercial pasteurized milk *also* undergoes homogenization. This includes the various skim, low-fat, non-fat, and long-life varieties.

As a result, millions of people all over the world are causing specific and life-long harm to their bodies as a result of consuming homogenized milk.

To defend homogenization the milk industry has an argument that goes like this:

'Homogenized milk is actually more easily digested rather than causing a problem. The tiny fat globules are digested, and they don't circulate intact in the bloodstream.'

Ironically, this statement is true. As explained in the chapter *The Lethal Effect of UHT Milk*, homogenization does indeed increase digestibility of milk. And furthermore, the tiny fat globules are indeed digested – they don't circulate intact in the bloodstream.

But here's the rub: by super-homogenizing UHT milk and making it more digestible, a greater amount of harmful substances enter the body to cause disease and illness. Milk would be healthier to consume if it was less digestible!

Apart from raw untreated milk, all types of organic milk sold commercially are homogenized. With UHT, the homogenization of milk is more intense and this applies to organic and nonorganic UHT milk.

For information about the harm caused by casein please see Appendix A. For information about how whey protein damages the brain see the chapter 'Brain Disease'. And for more information about the unhealthy aspects of UHT homogenization see Appendix D.

The lethal UHT Effect

As stated in the previous chapter, virtually all pasteurized milk is also homogenized, including all types of organic milk and UHT milk. Regular pasteurized milk is usually pasteurized first, followed by homogenization soon afterwards as part of one continuous flow process. But UHT milk is processed the other way round. The following table shows the differences between the two main types of milk in the world:

HTST pasteurizated milk ► *Regular pasteurized milk, normally requiring refrigeration.* **(Organic and nonorganic)**	Heat-pasteurized to between 72° - 75°C (161.6° - 167°F) depending on method used. Typically homogenized at about 63°C (145.5°F), at a pressure of 130 – 200 bar.
UHT (Long Life) milk ► *Not meant to require refrigeration until opened, up to 6 months shelf life at ambient temperature.* **(Organic and nonorganic)**	Heat-pasteurized to between 140.0°C – 150.0°C (284°F - 302°F), depending on UHT method used. Typically homogenized at about 75°C (167°F), at a pressure of 241 – 276 bar.

Sources: [1] Dairy Processing Handbook, published by Tetra Pak Processing Systems AB, S-221 86 Lund, Sweden, [2] Technical Bulletin – homogenizer operation in UHT plants, Ivensys APV, TB-82.

As you can see, UHT milk is pasteurized and homogenized much more intensely than HTST (regular pasteurized milk). Compared to HTST, The pasteurization temperature for UHT is about double, the homogenization temperature is about 20% higher, and the homogenization pressure is typically about 57% higher!

This has a dramatic effect on the fat globules in UHT milk, breaking them down into much smaller more compact globules. The size of fat globules is affected by the heat of pasteurization *and* by the pressure of homogenization.

Fat globule size [of homogenized milk] *decreased as heat treatment increased.*[108]

In general, the higher the homogenization pressure, the smaller the size of the particles.[122]

The higher the pressure and the more passes employed, the smaller was the average diameter of the casein micelles.[141]

As UHT milk is homogenized at a much higher temperature and pressure (compared to regular pasteurized milk), the fat globules in UHT are on average about half the size as shown in the following table (see next page):

Average Diameter of Milk-Fat Globule 1µm = 1micron = 1,000 nm (nanometers)	
Raw untreated milk ▶ (organic and nonorganic)	1000 – 10,000 nanometers. *Average dia.: 4,000 nm* (4.0µm)
HTST milk ▶ (regular pasteurized, homogenized milk, organic and nonorganic)	1000 – 2000 nanometers. *Average dia.: 1,500 nm* (1.5µm)
UHT (Long Life) milk ▶ (ultra homogenized & pasteurized milk, organic and nonorganic)	200 – 1000 nanometers. *Average dia.: 500 nm* (0.5µm). Note: Average dia. of semi-skinned UHT is about 700 nm (0.7µm).

Sources: [1] Technical Bulletin – homogenizer operation in UHT plants, Ivensys APV, TB-82, [2] Fox, P.F., *Fat Globules in Milk*, Elsevier Science, 2002, [3] Edgar Spreer, Milk and Dairy Product Technology, CRC Press, 1998.

This big difference in fat globule size has a major effect on human health. The much smaller size of UHT fat globules greatly increases their *total* surface area, making them more compact and evenly spread throughout the milk.

When you put several different ingredients into a saucepan and cook them, they will be thoroughly mixed. This is what happens with UHT milk. The proteins, fats, toxins and hormones are all thoroughly 'cooked', mixed and re-distributed throughout the milk.

More specifically, some toxins become attached to the micronized fat globules. Other toxins become attached to proteins, and these proteins are in turn attached to (stuck to) fat globules.

The hormone IGF-1 in dairy milk is contained in the membrane that surrounds the fat globules. Homogenization has the effect of shredding and breaking up the membranes, thus dispersing fragments of membranes throughout the milk. After homogenization, the membrane material and fatty acids coalesce back together into much smaller globules than before.

As there is insufficient membrane material to form new complete membranes around the milk-fat, the newly formed but ruptured fat globules are sealed and partly coated by clumps of casein molecules (referred to as 'casein micelles').

As a result, the IGF-1 hormones that were contained in the original bigger globule membranes end up being re-distributed into the membranes of the smaller globules. Remember: all this has happened *before* the milk is consumed.

But once the milk is consumed, the **Lethal Effect of UHT** processing is to send more harmfuls subtances into the body (compared to regular pasteurized milk) instead of being excreted.

This happens because with UHT, fat globules have a much greater *total* surface area to which toxins and other harmful subtances become attached. Digestion is simply a process by which food is converted into substances (good or bad) that can be absorbed through the lining of the intestine and into the body.

When milk is consumed, the proteins are broken down in the stomach and small intestine and the fat is combined with all other dietary fat, which is emulsified (held in solution) by bile components in the small intestine. The bile and lipase enzymes in the small intestine break the fat down to fatty acids and monoglycerides, which can then be transported across the intestinal mucosa and into the body. Any toxins, damaged proteins and other harmful substances that were not attached to the fat globules when the milk was consumed are more likely to be excreted instead of being absorbed into the body. Most toxins cannot go through the intestinal lining (i.e. be digested) unless they 'ride piggy-back' with fats or proteins.

Note: Lipase is an enzyme in milk that helps to break down fat. The body naturally produces the lipase enzymes. But many people may not have sufficient quantity of lipase, or an illness may inhibit the body from producing lipase. In any case those individuals are unable to digest lactose, which is the predominant sugar in milk. It is particularly important for such people to avoid the consumption of any kind of milk.

With UHT milk, a greater proportion of toxins and harmful substances are attached to fat globules (by virtue of their greater total surface area), making the harmful substances more likely to pass through the intestine wall to enter the body and the bloodstream instead of being excreted. The manner in which toxins, heavy metals, hormones, and proteins pass through the intestinal mucosa and into the body is a very well studied subject.

For class D metals, [heavy metals that are toxic such as mercury, lead, cadmium, and uranium] *high affinity for proteins and many other biological molecules makes it unlikely that their ions, except perhaps extremely transiently, can exist free in biological systems. Instead, the metals occur in complexes, bound to both high- and low-molecular-weight ligands. Transfer of metals across [intestinal] cell membranes, at least in vivo, therefore generally involves transfer of diffusible metal complexes.[135]*

A frequent observation indicates that uptake of a metal across a cell [intestine] membrane may involve more than one parallel mechanism. Separate processes clearly may coexist for transporting a particular metal into a cell.[136]

Many investigators have studied the transport of heavy metals across cell membranes...Intestinal absorption and pulmonary uptake are the major routes of metal entrance into the body of higher organisms. What clearly emerges from the work is that no one mechanism is likely to exist that can fully explain this process in all cells. Even in one cell type, separate and parallel transport processes have occasionally been observed for metals.... [Fat soluble] metals passively cross cell membranes.[135]

Ironically, what emerges from the research into UHT milk is that it is *more* digestible compared to regular pasteurized milk. This is bad news because it means that a greater amount of harmful substances are digested. The less digestible the milk the greater the amount of harmful substances that will be excreted.

- *During the processing of commercially sold milk, homogenization reduces fat droplet size and alters interface composition by adsorption of casein micelles mainly, and whey proteins. The structural consequences depend on the sequence of the homogenization and heat treatments. Regarding human health, homogenized milk seems more digestible than untreated milk.[137]*

- *The dairy* [milk processing plant] *heats the milk to either 145 F... or 161 F for at least 15 seconds. Either temperature combination kills pathogens bacteria in the milk. Pasteurization (as well as homogenization) also makes milk more digestible.*[138]

The greater the intensity of homogenization (such as in UHT milk) the greater the digestibility. This is so because the process of homogenization is akin to the process of digestion.

When milk is homogenized all particles are broken down to smaller sizes; equally, when milk is digested all particles are broken down to smaller sizes by the bile and by enzymes. When milk is homogenized, all particles are emulsified (held in a liquid suspension); equally, when milk is digested, all particles are emulsified by bile.

This is why your mother always told you to bite your food well! It is a known fact that when food is well masticated it is better digested. UHT processing goes a long way to preparing the milk solids for better digestion.

We must, of course, remember that homogenisation itself does not make milk-fat more digestible as the fat is digested by enzymes in the gut called lipases and this digestion process will occur naturally in the body when the lipases come into contact with the milk-fat. But the point here is that UHT processing makes more of the milk solids and micronized fat globules available to lipase digestion, and hence more easily digested.

Raw milk advocates may refute this by saying that the enzymes in milk make *raw* milk more digestible than any kind of *pasteurized* milk. This may be so, but this is a different matter. The point here is that

UHT milk (including organic UHT) is more digestible because the pasteurization and homogenization processes prepare the milk for easier digestion. Consequently, the heavy metals, harmful IGF-1 hormones, damaged whey proteins, toxins and other harmful substances that you find in all kinds of milk *are also more easily digested* instead of being excreted. If you absolutely must drink milk (we highly recommend that you avoid all milk) then regular pasteurized will give your body fewer amounts of harmful substances by virtue of being less digestible.

Some people may argue that the size of fat globules is irrelevant because whatever their size they are all broken down and hence they are all treated equally by the digestive system. While it is true that milk fat globules of all sizes face the same basic digestive process in the human body, the health consequences can be quite different.

UHT milk has the following four characteristics (compared to regular pasteurized milk):

1. **Smaller globules.** UHT fat globules are about half the size in terms of their diameter, hence there are many millions more of them.

2. **Smaller casein micelles more widely spread.** UHT fat globules present the digestive system with a much larger *total* globule surface area. This surface area is mostly covered in casein micelles, plus some whey proteins. This means that much more of the casein is stuck to fat globules instead of floating around loose in the milk liquid.

   With raw milk you have large clumps of casein molecules (called micelles) floating around. To be digested they have to be broken up into smaller and smaller pieces, until eventually individual casein molecules are broken down to amino acids which are absorbed into the body. Many of these casein micelles are not digested.

With pasteurized milk, more of the casein micelles (compared to raw milk) have been broken up into smaller micelles and sub-micelles, and they have stuck to (medical term: 'adsorbed to') the fat globules.

With UHT milk the same has happened but to a much greater extent: greater break-up of casein micelles, smaller size of casein particles, and more casein stuck to a greater number of fat globules. Remember that the much higher temperature of UHT pasteurization increases the amount of binding (sticking together) of various substances. This in turn greatly increases their likelihood of being absorbed into the body.

3. **Greater emulsification.** UHT fat globules are more emulsified than regular pasteurized milk by virtue of being smaller, thus making them easier and quicker to become digested and absorbed into the body.

4. **Greater proximity of toxins.** UHT fat globules are much more tightly packed together and consequently the toxins, damaged whey proteins, IGF-1 hormones, and other harmful substances carried by the globules will be in greater proximity.

As the fat globules and their cargo of substances are broken down by the digestive system, the closer proximity of the globules has the effect of increasing the amount of substances that are absorbed through the intestine instead of being excreted. Most substances cannot be absorbed through the lining of the intestine on their own – they do it by being bound with other substances (fatty acids, proteins, amino acids).

So although fat globules of all sizes face the same basic digestive processes, the effects of UHT processing combined with the smaller size of UHT fat globules, greatly affects how the milk is digested and how it affects health.

To summarize, the micronized fat globules created by homogenization are not absorbed into the body of a healthy person undigested. There is little evidence for this apart from *Leaky Gut Syndrome* (see the chapter 'Leaky Gut Syndrome'). But the micronized fat globules do act as a 'conveyor belt' to send toxins into the body. This happens because the fat globules and their cargo of harmful substances become more digestible and therefore more likely to enter the body instead of being excreted.

Once inside the body, most of these harmful substances are not killed off or neutralized – rather, they travel via the bloodstream to many parts of the body to cause illness and disease. The digestion process unwittingly brings these harmful substances into the body along with other nutrients.

Of course, it could be argued that we always receive some degree of harmful substances with just about any kind of food we care to eat. However, in such instances, most if not all harmful substances are excreted. But with UHT milk (organic and nonorganic) it is different: because of the unique nature of homogenization combined with the plethora of harmful substances found in milk, a significant amount of these substances enter the body to cause illness and disease.

The Lethal UHT Effect then, results in a higher number of fat globules and their harmful cargo being digested (compared to regular pasteurized milk) instead of being excreted. This in turn 'feeds' a higher amount of toxins and harmful substances into the body.

- *Microscopic examinations of the fat globules in UHT and conventionally processed products revealed that the UHT products had a **larger portion of smaller fat globules**.*[111]

- *For fresh [pasteurized] milk, diameters of 1.0 – 1.5 are sufficient to avoid creaming for a few days. For UHT milk and other long-life products, diameters of **0.2 – 0.7 um should be targeted**, which totally eliminates creaming.*[112]

- *Homogenization reduces fat droplet size and alters interface composition by adsorption of casein micelles mainly, and whey proteins. Regarding human health, homogenized milk seems **more digestible** than untreated milk.*[151]

- *Commercial milk is homogenized for the purpose of physical stability, thereby reducing fat droplet size and including caseins and some whey proteins at the droplet interface. This seems to result in a **better digestibility** than untreated milk.*[152]

- *Most fat digestion occurs in the small intestine. First, the fat globules must be broken into small sizes so enzymes can act. This emulsification is accomplished under the influence of bile, a secretion of the liver. Bile contains a large amount of bile salts, the main function of which is to make fat globules break down. **The smaller the fat particles, the better the digestion.**[153]

There is plenty of evidence to support the view that the heat of pasteurization causes milk solids to bind. The evidence shows that the greater the heat, the greater the binding – here are some extracts from the research:

- *High temperature heat processing causes changes in the physicochemical properties of milk proteins and minerals. The principal physicochemical changes in milk proteins and minerals caused by heating include: whey protein denaturation, interaction [binding] of denatured whey proteins with casein micelles...deposition [binding] of the heat-induced colloidal phosphate onto casein micelles...Heat and drying treatments of whey protein concentrates cause protein denaturation and aggregation [binding], resulting in loss of solubility and functionality.*[97]

- *For UHT milk samples, it was found that with increasing temperature, an increasing amount of whey protein was bound to casein micelles in [UHT] treated milk.*[84]

- *The effects of heat/lactose on casein have been investigated. Casein proteins have been shown to bind lactose in amounts ranging from 2% to 8% under different experimental conditions. At 95°C casein bound twice as much lactose as when heated at 52°C.*[96] *[UHT is pasteurized at 141°C].*

- *Heating milk to above 100°C causes lactose to combine irreversibly with milk proteins [casein]. This reduces the nutritional value of the milk.*[101]

- *The changes in milk fat globules...were examined. The effects of heat treatment of milk at 95 °C for 20 seconds, prior to evaporation, on fat globule size and the milk fat globule membrane (MFGM) proteins were also determined. In both non-preheated and preheated whole milk, the size of milk fat globules decreased while the amount of total surface proteins at the fat globules increased.*[104]

- *The effects of heat treatment and homogenization of whole milk on chemical changes in the milk fat globule membrane (MFGM) were investigated. Heating at 80 °C for 3–18 min caused an incorporation of whey proteins into MFGM, thus increasing the protein content of the membrane and decreasing the lipid [fat]. In contrast, homogenization caused an adsorption of caseins to the MFGM but no binding of whey proteins to the MFGM without heating.*[105]

- *The milk fat globule membrane (MFGM) itself is altered during thermal [heat] processing. Milk is usually agitated during heating...which may cause changes in globule size due to disruption or coalescence; significant disruption occurs during direct UHT processing. Heating per se to above 70 C denatures proteins.*[106]

In conclusion the much higher intensity of UHT homogenization and pasteurization causes a greater amount of smaller fat globules and a greater degree of binding of the various milk solids with fat globules. This results in a greater amount of harmful milk solids and toxins entering the bloodstream via the normal digestion process.

Because of this, UHT milk (including organic UHT) is worse for health than regular pasteurized milk. Milk consumers should note that the vast majority of organic milk production in the world is UHT and many milk products include UHT milk.

Here is a summary of the main points in this chapter:

- When UHT milk is homogenized it ruptures the fat globules and breaks them down to a much smaller size. So although pasteurized milk and UHT milk have similar amounts of total fat, UHT has a greater number of smaller fat globules.

- Smaller fat globules become more compact (because of their greater number) and more evenly spread throughout the milk. This puts the fat globules into closer proximity with the molecules of damaged milk solids and toxins that may be present.

- Then when the ultra high pasteurization temperature is applied immediately after homogenization, the milk solids, proteins and toxins in close proximity bind with the fat globules in the milk.

- Simultaneously, the ultra high heat serves to seal the ruptured globules by coating them with casein.

- By virtue of their smaller size and their casein coating a greater number of the UHT fat globules and their harmful cargo will be digested instead of being excreted.

- In the process of being digested, the toxins and harmful milk solids that were bound with UHT fat globules are released into the bloodstream. The harmful substances are then taken to many parts of the body (including the brain) to cause disease and illness.

- UHT milk (**including organic UHT**) is worse for health compared to pasteurized milk because it gives the body harmful substances on a greater scale, pint for pint.

Nutrition

The milk industry is a multi-billion dollar business. It spends millions of dollars promoting milk through many channels and at many levels. Because of this, unless you look below the surface, it is easy to be blinded by the belief that milk is nutritious and good for you.

The truth is that dairy milk has no redeeming features – all kinds of dairy milk are bad for human health.

Look at any milk carton and you will see a list of nutrients contained in milk. However, the reality is that very few of those nutrients end up benefiting the human body. This is so for three reasons:

1. Poor absorption.

In general, people who consume dairy milk cannot absorb vitamins and minerals as efficiently as people who don't. When your internal membranes and organs are congested with thick casein mucus, the body simply cannot absorb nutrients efficiently, and only a fraction of the nutrients will actually be absorbed and used by the body. In particular, the kidneys become congested with casein and this in turn prevents certain vitamins and minerals from being absorbed into the body.

In case you think this is an exaggeration, here is a scientific explanation. Casein from dairy milk has a tendency to coat the digestive organs of the body with unwelcome mucus (including the kidneys). Appendix A explains how the casein from milk enters the body to cause harm.

As a result, the kidneys do a poor job filtering the blood and keeping it clean. This in turn leads to poor ccll functionalily, in particular poorly cleaned blood affects oxygenation, and this prevents cells from absorbing fully the nutrients they need to stay healthy. When this happens, the cells do not communicate or work together properly (healthy cells are great team players!). The end result is disease, lethargy, and poor health.

Milk curdles immediately upon entering the stomach, so if there is other food present the curds coagulate around other food particles and insulate them from exposure to gastric juices, delaying digestion long enough to permit the onset of putrefaction. This reduces the efficiency of vitamin and mineral absorption from other foods being consumed at the time.

2. Nutritional loss.

- **Harmful protein.** As explained in *Appendix A*, with UHT more casein gets digested and consequently more of the harmful casein amino acids enter the body to cause harm. This results in mucus congestion that coats epithelial cells and interferes with efficient digestion of nutrients. Casein is a vitamin robber. This is what happens:

  ➢ When milk is consumed the casein protein is broken down to amino acids, some of which are digested into the body, and some are excreted.

  ➢ The amino acids from casein that are excreted are flushed out of the body, mostly through urine and sweat. But on the way out, the amino acid molecules become attached to molecules of magnesium, zinc, calcium and other nutrients, thus robbing the body of these valuable minerals.

> So even if some of the minerals in milk are absorbed, most will 'turn around' and leave the body. This does not happen with amino acids from plant-based food, because the human body is able to use all the amino acids, with little or no excess.

- **Heat treatment.** The pasteurization process involves heating milk to very high temperatures, serving to destroy much of its vaunted nutritional benefits.

The fact that the heating process kills all beneficial enzymes and many vitamins is not disputed, even by the milk industry. Organic UHT milk, which is heat-treated at about double the temperature of pasteurized milk, is even more devoid of nutritional benefits because more nutrients are destroyed by the heat or become bound with casein and leave the body.

The *'Dairy Processing Handbook'* readily admits that UHT milk *'is exposed to such powerful heat treatment that all relevant micro-organisms and most of the heat-resistant enzymes are inactivated.'*[117]

There is plenty of research showing that the very high temperatures of UHT greatly diminish the quality of nutrients in the milk:

- *Heating of milk can cleave* [bind] *the calcium phosphate complexes with casein micelles* [particles containing casein molecules and other substances], *resulting in destabilization.*[81]

- *UHT processing transfers minerals from the aqueous phase to the casein micelle and reduces ionic calcium levels by 10 to 20%. Some calcium phosphate is rendered insoluble at the high temperatures used in UHT heating. Losses of 20* and 30% respectively In thiamine and vitamin B12, can occur during UHT treatment. The levels of vitamin C and folic acid are markedly reduced.[84]

3. Medication. Dairy cows are heavily treated with hormones and antibiotics which are passed onto humans through the milk. Without medication, dairy cows would not be commercially viable. Medication is what enables cows to stay in an almost permanent state of lactation.

Antibiotics in particular have a dramatic effect in preventing vitamin absorption in humans: the antibiotics in pasteurized milk virtually cancel out many of the vitamins contained in the milk consumed.

For example, research has shown that vitamin K in dairy milk is hardly absorbed or used by the body because of antibiotics. As explained in the chapter 'Myths & Realities' both organic and nonorganic milk have antibiotics.

So coming back to the question: *'Is dairy milk a good source of nutrition?'* The answer is that although dairy milk contains some vitamins and minerals, these provide little nutritional benefit because they are mostly not absorbed, and because dairy milk (including organic milk) harms the body, acting as a nutrient robber.

Organic UHT milk provides even less nutritional benefit than regular pasteurized milk because of the higher temperatures used in UHT which serve to destroy its nutritional value. For more information on milk nutrition please see the chapter *'The More Nutritious Myth'* and also Appendix F.

Pesticides

When people buy organic milk, uppermost on their mind is the perception that the milk will have less or no pesticides compared to regular pasteurized milk. For many people this is the main reason they buy organic milk.

This perception is based on the assumption that organic cows are not fed with anything containing pesticides, whether the feed is grass or grain. The reality is that there is very little difference, if any, between organic and nonorganic milk when it comes to pesticides.

US Nutritionist Karen Collins, M.S., R.D., C.D.N. commenting on organic milk states the following:

'When evaluating the health claims, thus far, research does not support a health advantage of organic over conventional milk for any segment of the population. Recent USDA reports show that nonorganic milk may contain low levels of certain pesticides, but these are far below established tolerance levels. Using organic feed may support sustainable farming practices, yet research has not found it affects the nutritional value of the cows' milk.'

The USDA's Pesticide Data Program (PDP) is the most sophisticated government program in the world that tests food for pesticide residues. When milk was tested for pesticide residues in 1996, 1997, and 1998 very few residues were found.

In fact, only about 15 percent of the samples tested in each of those years had a single residue; about 85 percent of the samples contained no detectable residues. About 95 percent of the residues found were DDE, a breakdown product of the well-known chlorinated hydrocarbon insecticide DDT, which was banned from agricultural use in the early 1970s. DDT is very persistent and remains in many cropland soils.

In March 2008 The Organic Center (USA) issued a report stating the following:[159]

'Milk was tested for pesticide residues in 1996, 1997, and 1998 [and 2004]. Very few residues were found. In 2004, ten of the 739 samples of milk tested were reported as "organic". Just like virtually all samples, all 10 organic samples contained DPA and nine had DDE residues. DPA is a high volume industrial chemical used for many purposes in manufacturing rubber and plastic parts, and in making certain drugs. It is also a pesticide that is used as an apple plant growth regulator.

Of the 739 milk samples tested in 2004 by the USDA, 100% contained low level pesticide residue, all below actionable levels. The levels of DDE, DPA, and other pesticides found in milk in 2004 were very low. Most fell below one part per billion (ppb). The highest residue levels found were, at most, one-quarter of the applicable EPA tolerance (the maximum allowable limit of a pesticide in a given food).'

The Organic Center acts as a kind of shadow USDA, digesting the latest peer-reviewed research on organic food, translating it into English, and issuing summary reports.

Whether or not the levels of pesticides in milk are acceptable, *The Organic Center* report adds weight to the fact that there is little difference in pesticide levels between organic and nonorganic milk.

The report concludes that pesticide residues are in the body-fat of all Americans and most farm animals and wildlife. *Conventional and organic farmers can do little to avoid the DDE residues in milk.* Over the next thirty to fifty years these residues will gradually decline below limits of detection.

Although the latest USDA reports show that organic and nonorganic milk may contain low levels of certain pesticides, these are deemed to be below established tolerance levels. USDA regulations state that cow feed and pastures must not contain harmful pesticides. But the USDA gives no clear guidance on which pesticides are deemed harmful and which not, thus giving the *organic* farmer license to use pesticides at his discretion. As an aside, using so-called 'organic feed' may be said to support sustainable farming practices, yet USDA research has not found that it affects the nutritional value of the cows' milk one way or the other.

The exposure of organic crops to *synthetic* pesticides is, indeed, less than that of conventional crops, but crop growth results are somewhat variable and often misinterpreted. **USDA results from the *Pesticide Data Program* show no significant differences in pesticide levels between conventional and organic milk.**

A survey in Italy concluded that organic and conventional samples of milk do not show relevant differences for organochlorine pesticides, PCBs, and heavy metals. It should be pointed out that regulatory surveys worldwide do not test for organic pesticides – including non-synthetic and approved synthetic.

In a review conducted by Cal-Davis and IFT,[52] it was reported that organic milk contains less pesticide residue than conventional milk, but *'the marginal* benefits of reducing human exposure to pesticides in the diet through increased consumption of organic milk appear to be insignificant. It is important to consider the risks, if any, currently posed by pesticide residues in foods before determining the incremental health benefits from consuming organic products. Results on pesticide residues in organic vs. conventional milk and dairy products is mixed at best, and shows no clear advantage for consuming organic milk.'[1]

Many 'health' claims made by organic milk producers simply do not hold up to close scrutiny. Organic milk & dairy food advocates have been very aggressive in their advertising, promotion and sales using statements and "facts" that lack scientific validity. Some of this information may be true within a given context, but much is false and/or misleading.

Professor Rusty Bishop (Director, *Center for Dairy Research,* University of Wisconsin) states the following:

'Science does not support the health, nutrition, or safety claims made by the organic industry. Actually, toxin levels have been shown to be higher in organic foods [including organic milk] due to ineffective pesticide treatment of organic grain crops.'[1]

The U.S. Organic Trade Association, based in Massachusetts, USA, says that "Organic production is more environmentally sound because organic farmers are not using toxic and persistent synthetic pesticides that can remain in the air, water or soil for years to come." (Holly Givens, public-affairs manager).

But organic fertilizers and pesticides are not necessarily 'better' than synthetic equivalents. Organic fertilizers include agricultural and farmyard waste and animal sludge which greatly increases the amount of pathogens that come into contact with cows.

Some of these pathogens are not broken down by earthworms and insects in the soil, causing contamination and illness in cows, and even in milk consumers:

'Some kinds of bacteria in dairy milk are able to survive pasteurization, causing Johne's Disease, Crohns Disease, and IBS...'[6]

Indeed, most organic milk in the world is sold as UHT precisely because it is feared that mere pasteurization is not enough to make *organic milk* safe from pathogens.

There is a misconception that 'organic' means no pesticides. In fact, organic dairy farmers (just about anywhere in the world) are allowed to use a number of toxic chemical-pesticides, and many *organic* crops and pastures are routinely sprayed with toxic pesticides. For example, the use of rotenone is permitted in organic farming in America, Europe, and most other courtiers, yet rotenone is classified by the World Health Organisation as 'moderately hazardous' and capable of causing acute toxicity and death in humans.

The fundamental difference between organic and synthetic pesticides is not their toxicity, but their origin – whether they are extracted from 'natural' sources or chemically synthesized. In fact, some organic pesticides have toxic levels that are far higher than many synthetic pesticides.[115]

The most heavily used pesticide on organic farms is the toxin from the soil bacteria Bacillus thuringiensis, commonly referred to as 'Bt'. Although Bt is not thought to be harmful to mammals and birds, it does kill a vast range of insects, and this cannot be good for the environment.

Copper is a highly toxic heavy metal that is widely used as an organic fungicide. It is the 18th most used pesticide in the United States. Over thirteen million pounds of copper were applied to 54 crops in the USA in 1997.

So-called 'organic pastures' and cow-feed often contain high concentrations of copper and this is passed into milk. In the UK for example, the Soil Association recommends *copper oxychliride, copper ammonium nitrate, copper sulphate and soft soap* for use in organic production systems. Nearly a third of all UK organic farms used copper fungicides in 2006. (Source: soilassociation.org, published 1/3/2008).

The Soil Association states: *"If all UK farmland switched to organic, this would result in a 98% reduction in pesticide use."* It should be noted however, that although synthetic pesticide use would be reduced, organic pesticides would not. If anything, the use of organic pesticides would increase in the absence of synthetic pesticides, thus leading to more toxicity, more pressure on agricultural land, and more devastation of insect life and wildlife.

Copper fungicides and sprays are used in organic farming in all parts of the world and their use is increasing year on year.

'Agtrol, whose main interests are in copper fungicides, operates in 85 countries. Its sales in 2000 were US$50 million, according to Nufarm'.[150]

There are quite a number of other organic pesticides, including insecticidal botanical extracts such as pyrethrum, neem, and sabadilla, as well as insecticidal soaps and sprays such as kaolin, many of which are used in organic farming.

Surprisingly, government regulators have no statistics on the use of most organic pesticides. This is somewhat puzzling because many organic pesticides are used more intensively per acre than non-organic pesticides. This is due to the lower effectiveness of organic pesticides compared to their synthetic counterparts.

It has been estimated that if USA farming went entirely organic it would mean more pesticide use, not less; more toxicity, not less; and higher pressures on agricultural and other natural resources without any apparent offsetting benefits.[115]

The use of some organic pesticides for arable farming is to be applauded provided their use is monitored just as synthetic pesticide use is monitored, but this generally does not happen. It is wrong for organic dairy farmers to claim they 'do not use pesticides' or that their cow-feed is 'free of pesticides.' This is simply not true.

The crucial point here is that even though low levels of pesticides may be present in both organic and nonorganic milk, organic UHT milk will carry a higher proportion of the pesticides into the human blood stream.

This happens because with UHT milk more toxins are digested and less are excreted. For a fuller explanation see the chapter *The Lethal UHT Effect*.

In conclusion then, there is no significant difference in the level of pesticides in organic and nonorganic milk, which are in any event very low. However, a consumer of organic UHT milk is likely to absorb a higher amount of pesticides as a result of *The Lethal UHT Effect*.

Harmful Fat

Dairy milk contains saturated fat which is harmful to health. Organic and nonorganic milk are both high in saturated fat which is known to cause obesity, heart disease, cancer and many other diseases in the human body. There is little difference in fat between organic pasteurized milk and nonorganic pasteurized milk. But as you will see, there is a big difference between organic UHT milk and regular pasteurized milk.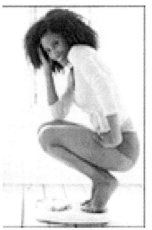

In addition to saturated fat, dairy milk contains trans-fats (trans-fatty acids) a type of fat which is even more harmful than saturated fat. Trans-fats are formed by *heating* fat or by *mixing air* into fat. This changes the molecular structure. Such fats are harmful to health because they clog up arteries and veins and in so doing contribute to a multitude of diseases. Unlike saturated fat, trans-fats are more difficult to get rid of: they penetrate more deeply into nooks and crannies of the body (including the brain).

UHT milk is higher in harmful trans-fats than non-UHT milk. This is so because the very high temperatures used for UHT serve to convert (i.e. hydrogenate) some of the milk fats into trans-fats. Milk producers may argue that the boiling point (saturation point) of fat is 200° C and UHT only goes to 141° C. However, it is known that hydrogenation is a gradual process that occurs as the fat is being heated up; it's not a case of reaching 200° C and then all of a sudden all the fat is converted into trans-fats. So when the milk is ultraheated at temperatures that reach 141° C, it is enough to convert some of the molecules in milk fat into harmful trans-fatty acids. (Note that here we are talking about harmful trans-fats, not the small amount of benign trans-fats in milk known as C18 monounsaturated trans-fatty acids).

Look at the label on a carton of milk in the USA (whether or not organic) and you will see that it says it contains a zero amount of trans-fatty acids (or it may not mention trans-fatty acids at all). In reality, all milk contains trans-fatty acids, but when the amount is below 0.5% per 100g of milk the authorities allow the labelling to show the amount as zero. This misrepresentation of trans-fats is further compounded by the similarity between the tiny homogenized fat globules and trans-fats, they are both equally harmful.

All dairy milk contains trans-fats, except non-fat milk. The level of trans-fats in dairy milk varies, depending on animal feeds, grazing, and other factors. In the USA and some other countries, there is no requirement to state the level of trans-fats on the label if the amount is not over 0.5g per 244g of fat. Consequently, no level of trans-fats is shown on milk carton labels. But the 0.5g threshold is often breached because levels of trans-fats vary considerably between 0.2g and 5.0g and random testing by the authorities, apart from being expensive and time consuming, is not enough to police the situation effectively.

In many countries, including the United Kingdom, there is no legal requirement at all to show the level of trans-fats in foods and on labels. This means that milk can be full of trans-fats and yet give no indication of this on the milk carton or container!

'Trans-fatty acid levels in dairy milk are quite high. Children should avoid trans-fatty acids as a matter of family policy, otherwise you are doing them a considerable disservice [at a critical time in their development]. One should restrict foods that contain trans-fatty acids'. Source: Dr. Michael Schmidt, author of 'Brain-Building Nutrition' and a world authority on nutritional medicine.

Acidity

The human body's chemistry is very sensitive to the level of acidity in the blood and cells. Acidity is measured by what is known as the pH scale, which runs from 0 pH to 14 pH. Below 7pH means higher acidity, and above 7pH means higher alkalinity.

Each pH point represents a ten-fold increase or decrease. For example, 5 pH is ten times *more* acidic than 6 pH.

Water at 7 pH is neutral, and the blood is on average 7.365 pH (slightly alkaline). Different areas of the body have different ideal pH levels.

> *Over-acidification of body fluids and tissues is a major cause of disease. It also weakens the immune system, making infection more likely and more severe.*[74]

In terms of the diet, no food is completely alkaline or completely acidic. But the body generally prefers alkaline food and dislikes acidic food. The more alkaline (and less acidic) the food you eat, the healthier you will be.[74]

Raw milk has an acidity rating of about 6.7 pH, which is slightly acidic. Pasteurized and UHT milk have an acidity rating of about 6.5 pH if measured straight after pasteurization, which is slightly more acidic than raw milk, but consider the following: many foods, such as meat, can have a low acidity rating, yet be highly acidic once consumed.

Once milk is consumed, it causes high acidity in the body (see Appendix A for a fuller explanation). Many studies corroborate this:

- Dr. Robert Young, author of the book 'The pH Miracle' states that 'When you eat acidic foods, the body tries to return to its alkaline state the only way it can – by withdrawing calcium from your bones...osteoporosis is a calcium-robbing problem, not a calcium–deficiency problem. Dairy milk is highly acid-forming. It can increase cancer risk. The idea that dairy products are healthy is pure hype – a cultural myth. Milk is full of components of no use to us, and they must either be converted to use (wasting our body's resources in the process) or eliminated as toxins.'[74]

- In the book 'Milk, dietary calcium, and bone fractures in women' the authors state: 'You should avoid too much protein. Consuming too much protein can leach calcium from your bones. As your body digests protein, it releases acids into the bloodstream, which the body neutralizes by drawing calcium from the bones. Animal protein seems to cause more of this calcium leaching than vegetable protein does.'[75]

UHT milk (including organic UHT milk) causes more acidity in the human body compared to regular pasteurized milk for two reasons:

I. It is well known that when animal protein is heated or cooked beyond a certain temperature acidity levels are increased. The higher pasteurization temperatures of UHT make the protein in milk more acidic.

  The process of pasteurization separates the milk from the friendly bacteria within it, which are killed by the heat. The acidity of pasteurized milk also increases to the point that it's no longer neutral.[78]

II. The longer the period of storage of UHT milk the more significant the increase in acidity. Here we are referring to the regular UHT cartons and plastic containers of milk that are stored until sold to consumers. Compared to nonorganic milk, UHT milk (including organic UHT) is stored significantly longer in the supply chain (warehousing, distribution, supermarket shelving, etc). For supporting evidence please see *Appendix E: Effects of UHT Storage.*

There have been reports that some stores are putting UHT milk out for sale when the expiry date is only about a week or so in the future. The fear is that if consumers see an expiry date that is, say 5 or 6 months hence, they will think the milk is 'too different' to regular pasteurized milk and not buy it. So if you see UHT milk with a date that is only one or two weeks hence, it means the milk is several months old and will have deteriorated even more than usual.

In conclusion, UHT milk (***including organic UHT***) causes more acidity in the body, and hence more illness. The greater acidity of UHT milk arises from two factors:

1. Casein in milk causes acidity (see Appendix A).

2. UHT milk deteriorates and become more acidic with storage (see Appendix E).

Brain Disease

Brain disease can be caused by a variety of factors such as the accumulation of heavy metals in the brain, alcoholism, faulty genes, malnutrition, and even lifestyle factors. But damaged proteins are generally regarded as one of the biggest causes of brain disease:

Protein misfolding [damaged proteins] *are increasingly recognized components of many neurodegenerative disorders.*[95]

What is a damaged protein? All proteins will "fold" into a specific, natural structure when left in water. A damaged protein is a misfolded protein. So a whey milk protein has a natural, specific structure technically referred to as the *nondenatured structure of whey protein.* By definition, a protein becomes denatured when its native structure is modified, even if only slightly modified. That's all that denaturation means - that the natural structure of the protein was somehow disrupted and that the protein has taken on a new structure, even if only slightly different.

Once a protein has become damaged (denatured) it becomes toxic to human health and can no longer be broken down into amino acids for use by the body.

What can cause denaturation of whey protein? Heat and acidity changes will cause whey protein to change structure. Once that structure change occurs, in chemical terms, the protein has become denatured.

'In the presence of heat, whey proteins denature, coprecipitate with casein and become insoluble... they too can be adsorbed onto the homogenized fat globule.' (Donna Gorski, 'Food scientists, don't forget about homogenization - milk processing' Dairy Foods, August, 1994).

'Whey protein can be denatured by heat. High heat, like the sustained high temperatures above 72 degrees Celsius associated with pasteurization, denatures whey proteins.' (Wilkipedia). Note: UHT milk is pasteurized at over 140°C.

Denaturation means that the protein has changed from its natural, native structure to some different, artificial structure. Once a protein has been denatured, the process cannot be reversed – the protein cannot be undenatured.

There is a common misconception that denatured protein is somehow better for you because it is 'more easily digested'. Nothing can be further from the truth. This misconception may have arisen from the way yogurt and some kinds of cheese are made. These products are often made by preheating the milk to temperatures high enough to denature the whey protein so that it acts as a gelling (coagulating) agent. But although denatured whey is used in making yogurt and cheese, it does not follow that it is healthy to eat.

In the distant past, yogurt and cheese were made from raw milk and with no heating processes involved – hence no denatured whey protein. Today, when making most kinds of commercial cheese with modern heating equipment, the damaged whey proteins are filtered out and what remains is a narrow range of non-damaged proteins that have survived the cheese manufacturing process. Eating yogurt and cheese containing denatured protein is as unhealthy as consuming milk with denatured whey protein.

The fact is, denatured (i.e. damaged) protein is common to all human neurodegenerative diseases, including Alzheimer's, Parkinson's, Lou Gehrig's and Huntington's Disease.

In the case of Huntington's Disease, a team of Northwestern University researchers discovered that the Huntington protein severely interferes with the function of the proteasome, the cellular process responsible for eliminating **damaged proteins** within the cell. The proteins that are normally broken down also build up within the cell. The researchers believe this information could help explain the disease process of Huntington's and perhaps other neurodegenerative diseases as well. The research was published in the October 27, 2004, issue of The EMBO Journal.

The astounding picture that is emerging is that damaged proteins severely interfere with the working of the proteasome, the cellular 'machine' responsible for eliminating damaged proteins within the cell. As a result, the build-up of toxic proteins escalates rapidly.[89]

The serious harm caused by consuming damaged whey proteins cannot be overemphasized, and since 2004, more and more research is coming to light proving this to be so.

It therefore bears repeating several times that misfolded (i.e. damaged) proteins are common to all human neurodegenerative diseases.

Lifestyle factors such as drinking, smoking, stress, and even environmental pollution can cause damaged proteins to build up in the human body. Just growing old can increase the build up of damaged proteins. But by far the biggest source of damaged proteins is the diet. And UHT milk contributes far more damaged proteins than any other food source.

In another major study published in January 2007 a clear link was found between Parkinson's Disease and milk. The diets of over 130,000 people were analysed and it was found that those who consumed the most cow's milk had a massive 70 percent higher risk of getting the disease.[99]

Furthermore, there is ample and growing evidence that protein misfolding (i.e. damaged or denatured protein) is at the root of many neurodegenerative disorders, not just the more serious diseases already mentioned. An in-depth examination of this subject is beyond the scope of this book – if you wish to find out more, a Google search for the following phrase provides over 23,000 results: *"protein misfolding" neurodegenerative*.

> *Drinking a glass or two of milk each day may increase the risk of Parkinson's disease later in life. The risk of Parkinson's disease increases as the amount of milk consumed each day goes up. Heavy milk drinkers were 2.3-times more likely to develop Parkinson's disease than non-milk drinkers.*
> Source: Neurology, April 2005.

Milk contains high concentrations of damaged whey proteins by virtue of the pasteurization and homogenization process. In particular, UHT organic and nonorganic milk is known to be high in damaged (denatured) whey proteins because of the very high pasteurization temperature:

- *Thirty-eight or more food factors are changed or destroyed* [by pasteurization], *including protein, enzymes, vitamins and minerals. Fats are also altered by the heat of pasteurization as well as the whole protein complex, which is rendered less available for tissue repair and rebuilding.*[59]

- *These changes in milk protein may be the result of sterilization of milk at very high temperature as the weight of casein micelles [molecule structures] increased with the severity of heat treatment.*[73]

- *UHT treatment of milk will cause denaturation of at least some of the heat-sensitive whey proteins. The direct heating process [UHT process] causes 60-70% denaturation.*[90]

- *Whey proteins will start to denature at temperatures in excess of 75°C. Considerable research has been done on whey proteins and [this research] has been used as a model system for understanding fouling in milk. Whey protein concentrates were found to be unstable to UHT processing.*[91]

- *More severe thermal [heat] treatment will increase protein denaturation, accompanied by loss of solubility and functional properties.*[98]

- *A decrease in whey protein levels is observed due to their partial denaturation… during the process of pasteurization. It has been fully proved and documented that pasteurization carried out under even "milder" conditions may cause irreversible thermal damage to the whey proteins. At 72°C whey is denatured by more than 60%. In the case of UHT, chromatographic evidence shows an additional dramatic decrease of [non-denatured] whey protein levels.*[92]

- *UHT treatment actually improves the digestibility of whey proteins.*[163] Ironically, improved digestibility is what you don't want because it means a greater amount of damaged and non-damaged whey proteins enter the bloodstream.

It is clear then that the high temperatures of the UHT pasteurization process serve to create damaged whey proteins that can increase the risk of brain disease. But the story does not end there.

As mentioned in this book (see Appendix E), UHT milk when stored for weeks or months before being consumed, is significantly more acidic than regular pasteurized milk. This acidity can damage whey proteins, in addition to those already damaged by ultra high temperature treatment.

When you add homogenization to the picture, UHT milk provides the perfect cocktail for brain disease: a high concentration of damaged whey proteins and toxins are delivered to the bloodstream courtesy of homogenization, and from the bloodstream the damaged proteins and toxins are taken to the brain where they become lodged to accumulate over time. For this reason alone, UHT milk (including organic UHT milk) should be avoided.

Leaky Gut Syndrome

Scientitsts have known for a long time that undigested elements of food can penetrate the intestine walls in a variety of ways and enter the bloodstream. This can happen from a poor diet, from old age, or because the intestines become damaged through poor health.[154]

When this happens a greater amount of harmful subtances penetrate the mucosa lining the intestine wall and enter the bloodstream – a condition that doctors refer to as 'leaky gut syndrome'.

This chapter explains how LGS (Leaky Gut Syndrome) plays an important role in the life of just about any milk consumer. If you ever consume milk you are urged to read this section for the sake of your health.

A full explanation of LGS is beyond the scope of this book. A lot of information about LGS is readily available on internet by doing a search for "Leaky Gut Syndrome."

The official definition of LGS is *'an increase in permeability of the intestinal mucosa to luminal macromolecules, antigens, and toxins associated with inflammatory degenerative and/or atrophic mucosa or lining'.*

Put more simply, large spaces develop between the cells of the intestine wall allowing bacteria, toxins and food to leak into the bloodstream. In a normal healthy person the small intestine behaves like a selective sieve allowing only the breakdown products of digestion into the bloodstream. Nutrients and well digested fats, proteins and starches are readily able to transfer through the wall of the intestine and enter into the bloodstream whilst large molecules, microbes and toxins are kept out and are excreted from the body.

Some doctors dispute the existence of LGS claiming that it is unproven 'alternative medicine'. Scepticism about LGS arises because it is difficult to diagnose the condition as the *cause* of an illness. Straightforward urine tests exist which show whether there is any degree of intestinal permeability. But it is more difficult to prove any connection between intestinal permeability and a particular illness, hence the scepticism.

The concept of increased gut permeability itself is well recognised in various conditions, such as hepatic encephalopathy. So although experts may differ on the causes of LGS (candida, antibiotics, bacterial infections, chemotherapy, poor diet, gluten grains) leaky gut is generally no longer considered "alternative medicine" (Wikipedia).

LGS and food allergies often co-exist. That is, food allergies can increase intestinal permeability, causing an immune response and provoking further inflammatory reactions throughout the body. For example, most people are allergic to milk, and symptoms can vary greatly from mild discomfort to serious illness. Milk allergy is caused by the body's reaction to some of the proteins in dairy milk which cannot be fully digested.

Over time, dairy milk proteins will increase intestinal permeability causing the intestine to develop leakages that allow bigger molecules and undigested substances (referred to as "toxins") to pass through into the bloodstream. These toxins are passed onto the liver to deal with but it cannot cope with the overwhelming toxins and stores them in the body tissues to 'come back to' later on.

With a regular milk consumer, the liver becomes too overworked to 'go back' to the toxins and as the intestinal lining gets consistently weaker, more and more toxins and undigested food enter into the bloodstream. The immune system sends out antibodies to fight these foreign substances and in doing so, toxic oxidants are produced which attack the body tissues causing allergic reactions, pain and inflammation throughout the body.

Just about anybody who consumes dairy milk on a regular basis will gradually develop greater intestinal permeability leading to LGS. A healthy individual would have a strong enough immune system to control the leakage of toxic substances but as it becomes overloaded the toxins leak into the liver resulting in an overworked overburdened liver.

Milk is known to be one of the biggest dietary causes of LGS mainly because the protein casein acts to irritate the mucosa lining of the intestine. It does this because not all casein is broken down to amino acids. The left over casein micelles (clumps of casein molecules) scrape along the intestine on their way out of the body. In doing so, they irritate the delicate mucosa lining.

When milk is homogenized and pasteurized, whey proteins bind with casein proteins, and the casein in turn sticks to the surface of fat globules, virtually coating them.

This occurs following homogenization because changes in surface tension between the newly created fat globules and the surrounding milk liquid causes casein micelles (clumps of casein molecules) to stick to the fat globules and seal their ruptures to make up for any missing globule membrane material.[132] This is how whey and casein proteins end up coating the micronized fat globules.

UHT milk is worse for LGS because it presents a much bigger 'offering' of proteins to the digestive system. This is so because the fat globules in UHT milk are about half the size compared to regular pasteurized milk. This means the total surface area of fat globules in UHT is about double, and since fat globules are coated in proteins, the allergenicity caused by UHT is worse.

To clarify further, the total amount and variety of proteins is the same in both types of milk, the problem lies with the way the proteins are presented to the intestinal wall. With UHT, the intestine walls are more intensely covered by the milk proteins simply because of a greater presence of smaller micronized fat globules coated in protein.

Worse still, in a person suffering from LGS, some of the UHT fat globules are able to pass through the intestine wall *undigested*. Normally, UHT fat globules would be too big to pass through the intestine wall undigested, but as a person develops LGS, small gaps develop between cells in the intestine wall. With time these gaps become bigger until eventually the smaller UHT fat globules are able to penetrate through the wall and hence escape being broken down by the digestive system.

When UHT fat globules penetrate the intestine wall and enter the bloodstream they can be carried to many parts of the body. As they dissolve, their cargo of harmful proteins, cancer-causing hormones, heavy metals, and other toxins are left inside the body to cause disease and illness.

We have seen in the chapter *'The Lethal Effect of UHT'* that most fat globules in regular pasteurized milk have a diameter of at least 1,500 nanometers; this is usually too big to penetrate the intestine of a person with LGS. But fat globules in UHT milk vary in diameter between 200 and 1000 nanometers, and many of the smaller globules would be small enough to penetrate the intestine wall (without being digested) in a person with LGS. Here is some of the research:

- *Homogenization of milk breaks up the fat globules… and increases the number of globules about 100 times. These fat globules or liposomes can pass through the intestinal barrier and by way of the lymph stream, subclavian vein, right heart, pulmonary circulation, and left heart, can enter the aorta and general circulation.*[129]

- According to Lee Dexter, microbiologist from Austin, Texas, ultra-pasteurization is an extremely harmful process to inflict on the 'fragile' components of milk. Dexter explains that milk proteins are complex, three-dimensional molecules, like tinker toys: *'They are broken down and digested when special enzymes fit into the parts that stick out. Rapid heat treatments like pasteurization, and especially ultra-pasteurization, actually flatten the molecules so the enzymes cannot do their work. If such proteins **pass into the bloodstream** (a frequent occurrence in those suffering from "leaky gut,") the body perceives them as foreign proteins and mounts an immune response. That means a chronically overstressed immune system and much less energy available for growth and repair.*[118]

- *Once intestinal permeability has occurred, the body can easily become oversensitized, perhaps even allergic to certain foods due to the body's inability at the level of the intestine or the liver to completely breakdown these foods into usable components, hence they drift into our bloodstream and act as irritants. They may be culprits in causing migraines, eczema, rheumatoid arthritis, Crohn's disease and hyperactivity.*[139]

- *Cow milk is one of the most common food allergies. This may be due to homogenization, which may encapsulate small milk proteins in a molecular layer of fat, making them easier to leak out into the bloodstream, where they are attacked as germs. Over time an allergic reaction develops. If [a person] continues to drink milk, and it is an allergic irritant, it will continue to irritate the gut lining and prevent healing of the intestines, and prolong a Leaky Gut Syndrome.*[140]

Dr. Patina Muhammad, USA,[103] John McDougal MD, John Robbins (health book author), and others have reported how milk homogenization has an impact on health in several ways. Here are some of their comments:

- *Normally, large milk fat globules cannot penetrate the intestinal walls or arteries to enter the bloodstream. Homogenization transforms them into microscopic spheres of fat, which can then penetrate the walls of blood vessels, and as a consequence enter the bloodstream to be taken to all parts of the body.*

- *When in the bloodstream, the fat globules attack the plasminogen tissue of the walls of the arteries and parts of the heart muscle. (Plasminogen is a plasma protein that is found in the bloodstream.) This causes lesions in the arteries and heart muscle. Lesions are scratches, lacerations, abrasions, wounds or injuries.*

- *The body tries to heal itself by laying down a protective layer of cholesterol to prevent further damage. This then leads to scar tissue and calcified plaque and a build-up of cholesterol and other fatty deposits. Too much cholesterol in the blood vessels may lead to hardening of the arteries, heart disease, chest pains, and heart attacks. Even young children in the United States are showing signs of hardening of the arteries.*

Who is affected by LGS? In short, most people have a leaky gut, but in many people it is not sufficiently severe to be noticed as such.

LGS is caused my many factors: diet, age, lifestyle, medication, alcohol, stress, and other factors can all affect the gaps between cells in the small intestine. Any cursory investigation into LGS quickly reveals that dairy milk is one of the main dietary causes.

More than half the adult human population is likely to have some degree of leakage through the intestine. This means that many people who consume UHT milk are at risk of absorbing undigested milk fat globules and their cargo of harmful substances.

In conclusion, UHT milk (**both organic and nonorganic**) increases the risk of Leaky Gut Syndrome. This in turn increases the risk of absorbing undigested milk fat globules (and undigested substances from other food sources) into the bloodstream. And this in turn increases the risk of disease and illness as a result of harmful substances being brought into the body without being digested. Dairy milk, and UHT milk in particular, is a major contributor to Leaky Gut Syndrome.

Bovine Sex Hormones

Like IGF-1, bovine sex hormones can be found in all types of dairy milk. Here we are referring to estrogen and progesterone which are natural components of cow's milk, by virtue of pregnancy and lactation.

As explained in the chapter '*UHT and Cancer*', milk is rich in IGF-1 hormones which enter the body when milk is consumed. Equally, bovine sex hormones are naturally present in all dairy milk and will enter the body every time milk is consumed.

The sex hormones estrogen and progesterone are naturally bound with fat globules in milk. When milk is digested the sex hormones pass into the body and the bloodstream.

As explained in the chapter '*The Lethal UHT Effect*' UHT processing ensures that a greater amount of smaller fat globules are created. This in turn ensures that a greater amount of fat globules are digested, thus giving the body more bovine sex hormones compared to regular pasteurized milk.

So both organic and nonorganic UHT milk will deliver a higher percentage of sex hormones into the body compared to regular milk.

Bovine sex hormones are bad for both women and men by increasing the risk of cancer. For women, bovine sex hormones increase the risk of breast cancer by suppressing their progesterone. This happens because bovine sex hormones interfere with a woman's body chemistry. (Women produce varying levels of progesterone throughout their lives, whether or not pregnant, as it is so vital for life).

Furthermore, dairy milk interferes with the production of oxytocin in the woman's body. The hormone oxytocin is known to protect against breast cancer, yet another reason for avoiding dairy milk.[51]

For men, bovine sex hormones are known to cause testicular cancer and infertility, and have a feminizing effect on the body. Men do not require progesterone as it is a female sex hormone. Nevertheless, bovine sex hormones can also interfere with a man's body chemistry, possibly increasing the risk of various types of cancer.

· *Milk and dairy products [organic and nonorganic] contain the female sex hormones estrogen and progesterone. It is reasonable to hypothesize that estrogens or progesterone in milk and dairy products may be associated with the development of testicular cancer.*[26]

· *Dairy farming involves milking the cows even when pregnant, and this practice is associated with higher levels of estrogen and progesterone in milk, which in turn may increase risk of premature sexual development [in humans] and also breast cancer.*[27]

· *There are several reasons why dairy products raise a woman's hormone levels, causing a variety of hormone-dependent problems from early onset of menstruation (menarche) to PMS and uterine fibroids - but one is unique to cow's milk: cows are milked even while they are pregnant. As a result of the pregnancy, cows secrete high levels of estrogen into their milk.*[28]

The following edited extract is taken from the website www.notmilk.com:

Why is it that nations with the lowest rates of testicular and prostate cancers (Korea, Vietnam, Algeria, China) also have the lowest rates of dairy consumption? Why is it that the nations consuming the most cheese have the highest rates of testicular cancer?

Testicular cancer is the most frequently diagnosed cancer among North American males between the ages of 15 and 40.

According to the Testicular Cancer Research Center (TCRC.org), the nation with the highest rate of testicular cancer is Denmark, followed by Switzerland. Denmark and Switzerland also enjoy (?) the world's highest per capita consumption of cheese.

The October 10, 2003 issue of the International Journal of Cancer reveals that a high intake of cheese is associated with an elevated risk of testicular cancer in Canadian males.

University of Ottawa scientist Michael J. Garner (Department of Epidemiology and Community Medicine) compared the diets of 601 men who were diagnosed with testicular cancer to 744 controls.

According to the scientists, the results suggest: "...high dairy product intake, in particular high intake of cheese is associated with an elevated risk of testicular cancer in Canadian males."

In 2002, the International Journal of Cancer (Ganmaa, et al, 98:262-267) reported that diet has an important influence on testicular and prostate cancer risk. The study stated:

"Cheese was found to be most closely correlated with the incidence of testicular cancer. The incidence rate of prostatic cancer was highest in the U.S. followed by Canada, Iceland and Sweden" [all top milk-consuming countries].

Galactose

A type of sugar, galactose is found in small amounts in many foods, including fruit and vegetables. Dairy milk, however, is super-rich in galactose. Weight for weight, dairy milk typically has 20 to 30 times more galactose than, say, cheddar cheese or lentils, and 500 times more than an orange. For a list of foods showing their galactose content go to www.galactosemia.org.

The human body can use galactose in small amounts by converting it into energy. But the *very large* amounts provided by dairy milk cannot be broken down and used as energy and are toxic. The large surplus amounts of galactose provided by dairy milk end up causing illness in several ways. Note that here we are not talking about people allergic to galactose – people allergic to galactose can actually die from consuming dairy milk or any galactose rich food. **Galactose-rich dairy milk is bad for anybody, whether or not allergic to galactose!**

Several studies show that galactose from dairy milk increases the risk of cataracts in the eyes:

• *This patient presented with cataracts and galactosuria that developed upon drinking milk…The mechanism that produces galactose-related* **cataracts** *is understood fairly well…Diet is the foundation of therapy. Elimination of lactose and galactose sources suffices for definitive therapy.*[85]

• *Galactose is toxic in high doses or if insufficiently removed, and causes tissue damage above certain levels in humans. Galactose reaches high levels in human plasma following milk ingestion. Galactose increases atheromatous plaque formation in Baboons and other experimental animals, causes cataracts in rats (and possibly in humans), and is related to the onset of diabetes in humans.*[86]

Another study shows a strong link between galactose and infertility in women, caused by ovarian failure. The study concludes that galactose may be a precursor to ovarian cancer.[49] Many other studies show a close association between galactose and a variety of diseases, arising from dairy milk consumption. Doctors even have a name for galactose when it causes disease: *galactosemia.*

The dairy industry tries to solve the problem of galactose by marketing lactose-reduced milk. Unfortunately, such milk only encourages a greater consumption of a product that is unhealthy in many other ways. Note that compared to whole milk (i.e. regular 3% milk), evaporated milk contains twice as much galactose, and most goat's milk has about 10% more.

When it comes to organic UHT milk, research shows that UHT provides a higher amount of harmful galactose (compared to regular pasteurized milk) for two reasons:

1. UHT binds a higher amount of lactose to casein (which in turn is bound with fat globules). Casein then carries the lactose into the small intestine for digestion and absorption into the body. Lactose is water soluble, and since galactose is a component of lactose, the galactose gets distributed to many parts of the body by the bloodstream.

- *The effects of heat/lactose on casein have been investigated. Casein proteins have been shown to bind lactose in amounts ranging from 2% to 8% under different experimental conditions. At 95°C casein bound twice as much lactose as when heated at 52°C.*[96] [UHT is pasteurized at 141°C].

- *Heating milk to above 100°C causes lactose to combine irreversibly with the milk proteins [casein]. This reduces the nutritional value of the milk.*[101]

2. UHT milk is typically stored for several weeks (without refrigeration) before being opened or purchased by a consumer. Research shows that galactose content of UHT milk increases dramatically during storage, particularly if not refrigerated until sold (see Appendix E).

In his book *Milk and mortality*[50] Dr. David Gordon lists dozens of studies showing strong associations between galactose from dairy milk and disease.

Pus

How does a cow make milk? A dairy cow filters 10,000 quarts (about 11,000 litres) of blood through her udder each day and uses dead white blood cells to manufacture her milk. Put another way, dairy milk is mainly pus with hormones, and just about every cupful of pasteurized dairy milk contains pus. Humans make breast milk differently – the hormone prolactin makes the breasts produce milk.

The milk industry tries to argue that pus in milk (euphemistically referred to as *somatic cells*) is not harmful to humans, but the evidence contradicts this.

It is estimated that about one-third of cows being milked at any one time are stressed and infected. Milk from these cows contains large amounts of bacteria, viruses, and pus. As a consequence, farmers must treat their herds with increased amounts of antibiotics. In an extensive study, Pam Ruegg, a University of Wisconsin mastitis researcher, examined more than a million records, and concluded that the higher the herd's pus cell count, the greater the risk of antibiotic residues in milk. So pus goes hand in hand with antibiotics which are not neutralized by the pasteurization process.

Any lactating mammal excretes toxins through her milk. This includes antibiotics, pesticides, chemicals and hormones. Also, all cow's milk contains blood! The [US] inspectors are simply asked to keep it under certain limits. You may be horrified to learn that the USDA allows milk to contain from one million to one and a half million pus cells per milliliter (1/30 of an ounce).[9]

The dairy industry knows that there is a problem with pus in milk. Accordingly, it has developed a system known as the "somatic cell count" to measure the amount of pus in milk. The somatic cell count is the standard used to gauge milk quality. The higher the somatic cell count, the more pus can be found in the milk.

Any milk with a somatic cell count higher than 200 million per litre should not enter the human food supply, according to the American Dairy Association. Therefore, anyone living in a region where the somatic cell count is higher than 200 million shouldn't be drinking milk. There is only one problem— virtually every state in the USA is producing milk with pus levels so high that it shouldn't enter the human food supply! Even the US national average, at 322 million, is well above the industry's limit.

What about organic milk? Research carried out by Professor Rusty Bishop, Director of the *Center for Dairy Research*, Department of Food Science, University of Wisconsin, USA, shows that **organic milk is significantly higher in pus than nonorganic milk**. His research (see table on next page) shows the composition of data from '*130 midwest dairy farms, showing a major difference in rolling herds averages (RHA), slight but insignificant differences in fat and protein content of organic vs. conventional raw milk, and a somewhat significant difference in somatic cell counts (SCC).'*

See table on next page ▶

Gross compositional comparison of conventional vs. organic raw milk (n=130)

Milk	RHA	% Fat	% Protein	SCC
Conventional	24,676	3.83	3.06	236K
Organic	16,823	3.87	3.10	276K

(Source: *Science Behind Reported Benefits of Organic Milk,* October 12, 2007, Rusty Bishop, Ph.D., Director, Center for Dairy Research, Professor, Department of Food Science, University of Wisconsin – Madison, USA)

The above table shows that in this particular study organic milk had 17% more pus cells (Somatic Cell Counts) than nonorganic milk, a very significant difference! It is thought that organic cows generally have a higher somatic cell count – the reasoning for this goes as follows.

- A dairy cow (whether or not organic) must be kept in an almost continuous state of milk production to be commercially viable. Because of this, a cow will inevitably develop mastitis unless *routinely* given antibiotics. Organic cows cannot be given antibiotics *routinely*, only sporadically, at the farmer's discretion when he thinks the cow may need antibiotics for 'medical' reasons.

- Consequently, the organic farmer is caught between a rock and a hard place when it comes to pus in milk: he cannot give antibiotics *routinely* as a way of keeping the somatic cell count under control (otherwise he loses his 'organic' certification). But if he gives antibiotics sporadically instead of *routinely*, the somatic cell count will not abate. So to remain organic, a higher amount of pus in milk is an inevitable compromise.

- *Organic cow's milk is loaded with as much saturated fat and cholesterol as regular milk, and it is often contaminated with pus and blood from cows who had udder infections and weren't given medicine because, if they were, the farmers wouldn't be able to label their milk organic. The dairy herd is sick—these are sick and diseased cows, producing pus-filled milk that even industry standards call 'unhealthy.'*[126]

- *The somatic cell score continued to rise after 6 years of organic production. The higher somatic cell scores on organic farms agreed with many other studies (Kristensen and Mogensen, 1998; Vaarst et al, 2003; Smolders and Baars, 2004). We found the somatic cell scores did not stabilize after some years, but kept increasing for 6 years after conversion.*[125]

- *Similarly to what was found in Ontario [Canada], a study in Norway, comparing 31 organic and 93 conventional dairy herds, found higher somatic cell counts in organic farms.*[127]

- *'Somatic cell counts (SCC) are higher than 400,000 in 40% of the [organic] herds...'*[134]

Naturally, one cannot say that all organic milk has more pus than nonorganic, but it does mean it cannot generally be claimed that organic milk has a lower pus count.

Lactose Intolerance

Both organic and nonorganic milk contain sugar (i.e. carbohydrate) in the form of lactose. This lactose is broken down by the body into glucose and galactose. Unfortunately, all humans are lactose-intolerant, it's just a matter of degree. That is, all humans break down lactose with varying degrees of success

When someone is said to be *lactose-intolerant* it means the digestive system is not able to completely break down the lactose sugar in the milk. This inability results from a shortage of the enzyme *lactase*, which is produced by the cells that line the small intestine. As we become older, we produce less lactase, and therefore become more lactose-intolerant. That is why the elderly instinctively shy away from dairy milk.

It is natural to lose the lactase activity in the gastrointestinal tract. It is a biological accompaniment of growing up. Most people do it. All animals do it. It reflects the fact that nature never intended lactose-containing foods, such as milk, to be consumed after the normal weaning period.[58]

Persons of all races are affected by lactose intolerance, with higher prevalence among Asian, African, and South American people. In the USA the prevalence of lactose intolerance varies according to race. As many as 25% of the white population (prevalence in those from southern European roots) is estimated to have lactose intolerance, while among black, Native American, and Asian American populations, prevalence is estimated at 75-90%. Generally, 75% of the world's population is estimated to be lactose-intolerant. It is least common in races descended from northern Europe or from the north-western Indian subcontinent

Males and females are affected equally. However, according to some research, about 44% of women who are lactose-intolerant temporarily regain the ability to digest lactose during pregnancy. This is probably due to slow intestinal transit and bacterial adaptation during pregnancy. It is not a signal that dairy milk should be consumed!

Although lactose intolerance is a very common disorder that is present in many people, it is often ignored because it goes unrecognized. Symptoms of lactose intolerance include lose stools, abdominal bloating and pain, flatulence, nausea, and abdominal gurgling. To test yourself for lactose intolerance, see whether you have wind or a feeling of bloating within 5 - 30 minutes of consuming dairy milk.

A major problem is that people who suffer from lactose intolerance do not realize that it is being caused by dairy products (milk in particular is usually not suspected). Many times babies and toddlers suffer from wind and colic. The cause of all the pain, crying and distress on both the child and the parents may be the inability of the child to break down lactose. The fermentation of lactose in the bowels causes the formation of gases, including methane and carbon dioxide. These will cause the baby's intestines to inflate, causing pain and distress for all concerned. Unfortunately, doctors often find it difficult to pinpoint the presence of lactose intolerance and people with this condition are often wrongly classified as suffering from Irritable Bowel Syndrome (IBS).

As mentioned, we are, in fact, all lactose-intolerant to a degree. Some people suffer severely from it, while others experience very mild symptoms of discomfort. This is so because people produce different amounts of lactase in the small intestine. For example John may be producing just enough lactase to cope with a glass of milk in the morning before suffering any ill-effects, while Jane is not even able to have a lick of ice-cream without distress. The sad thing about lactose intolerance is that millions of people who consume dairy milk will suffer needlessly from its symptoms and make no association between the two, thus impairing their daily lives and well being.

Organic UHT milk provides the body with more lactose than regular pasteurized milk. This is so because, as explained in Appendix D, the higher temperatures of UHT combined with the effect of homogenization serve to bind a greater amount of lactose with casein/fat globules in the milk. This then gets absorbed into the body rather than being excreted.

- *The effects of heat/lactose on casein have been investigated. Casein proteins have been shown to bind lactose in amounts ranging from 2% to 8% under different experimental conditions. At 95°C casein bound twice as much lactose as when heated at 52°C.*[96] [UHT is pasteurized at 141°C].

- *Heating milk to above 100°C causes lactose to combine irreversibly with the milk proteins* [casein]. *This reduces the nutritional value of the milk.*[101]

So although UHT and non-UHT milk may contain similar amounts of lactose and casein, UHT milk (***including organic UHT***) gives the body a higher amount of lactose and casein that enter the bloodstream to cause harm.

Osteoporosis

Dairy milk (whether or not organic), far from protecting your bones, actually *causes* osteoporosis. This happens because milk causes valuable bone-making cells to wear out, thus increasing the risk of osteoporosis. It is a myth that the calcium in milk helps strengthen bones. All the recent research into this subject is showing the opposite to be the case, but such research tends to be drowned out by the enormous milk marketing industry and their lobbyists.

Organic UHT milk is worse for bones compared to regular pasteurized milk because UHT is more acid-forming once consumed (see 'Acidity' chapter). High acidity combined with high calcium causes an excess of calcium in the bloodstream – as a consequence, more bone-making cells become eroded, thus increasing the risk of osteoporosis.

For a fuller explanation please see *The Milk Imperative* at: www.milkimperative.com.

Calcification

Dairy milk (whether or not organic) causes harmful calcification, the biggest cause of illness in the world today.

All the latest research is revealing that in fact, calcification is responsible for more deaths through illness than anything else.[73] Here is a list of some of the diseases caused by calcification:

Diseases caused by harmful calcification

Aging skin	Macular degeneration
Alzheimer's	Multiple sclerosis
Arthritis	Prostatitis
Bone spurs	Psoriasis
calcification	Kidney Stones
Bursitis	Scleroderma
Cataracts	Stroke
Diabetes, type 2	Tendinitis
Liver cysts	Heart disease
Gallstones	Kidney stones
Glaucoma	Various types of cancer

Source: Mulhall and Hansen, The Calcium Bomb,
The Writers Collective,
2005, ISBN 1594111014.

Both organic and nonorganic milk cause harmful calcification because they both have high levels of calcium combined with high acidity. The high acid-forming propensity of milk combined with the high calcium content is a lethal cocktail tailor-made to cause harmful calcification.

Breast and prostate cancer in particular are caused by metabolic acidity combined with harmful calcification. For the evidence that milk is a major contributor to harmful calcification please see *The Milk Imperative,* (www.milkimperative.com).

Milk provides a perfect cocktail of ingredients for the development of cancer in the body of a milk consumer: acid forming casein, calcium and saturated fat.

Organic UHT milk causes more harmful calcification than regular pasteurized milk because UHT is more acidic (see 'Acidity' chapter). High acidity combined with high calcium greatly increases the risk of cancerous tumours in the body.

Myths & Realities

The Organic Standards Myth

Myth: Organic milk is based on recognized standards set by the 'organic industry'.

Reality: There are no organic milk standards.

There is no internationally agreed standard for organic milk, let alone national standards. For starters, nobody can agree what is meant by 'organic milk'.

In the USA, for example, there is a heated debate on this subject, with lawsuits flying in all directions. At the time of writing this report, lawsuits have been issued against US 'Aurora Organic Dairy' saying it has failed to meet federal organic standards. The U.S. Department of Agriculture has four requirements to define milk as organic, and confusion abounds about each.

It is important to understand that if a food product is certified "organic", this describes the process by which the food product was supposed to be produced and processed; it does not describe the product itself. The most controversial of these parameters is the "access to pasture" due to its vague meaning and its apparent abuse. There remain issues with international consistency of organic standards, especially from countries exporting organic products and ingredients to the U.S. For example, EU organic standards allow limited use of antibiotics. Critics claim China's fledgling organic industry is plagued by lax standards, inadequate oversight, exploitation of workers, and practices such as using human waste to fertilize fields, which isn't the kind of "organic" the USDA and most consumers support.[1]

Another issue is the conflict that exists among organic farmers themselves. On one side of the divide are those who believe that "organic" means small farms, often run by families. On the other side are those who say the only way to satisfy the growing demand is by applying industrial farming practices to organic milk production.

When it comes to standards in the European Union the situation is as confusing as North America. Quite simply, there is no set standard for organic milk.

In the United Kingdom, DEFRA (Department for Environment, Food and Rural Affairs) is responsible for regulations governing the production of organic foods and the administration of organic schemes. Their website states: *'All organic food must meet a common set of minimum standards that are set out in European law.'*

But although various bodies set standards for the organic farming of *animals*, there is nothing in the regulations that is specific to organic milk. In the UK there are over ten different bodies (associations, cooperatives, etc.) that vie for the position of being the certifying body for organic milk!

Here is a typical statement from one such body:

'Organic milk comes from cows that are not fed antibiotics and synthetic pesticides. It has all the nutritional goodness of nonorganic milk but, due to the cows' more natural diet, it also has some additional health benefits. Nonorganic milk comes from farms that are allowed to use GM cattle feed, routine antibiotic treatments and synthetic pesticides. These are not permitted on organic farms. In contrast, organic farmers use traditional methods to

produce purer, more natural organic milk that is good for you, the cows and the countryside.'

Let's briefly analyse this statement by breaking it down to four sections:

1. *'Organic milk comes from cows that are not fed antibiotics and synthetic pesticides.'* This is not so because organic cows are indeed given antibiotics when needed (this point is discussed later on).

2. *'...it also has some additional health* benefits.' What additional health benefits? As explained in this book, organic milk offers no health benefits compared to regular pasteurized milk.

3. *'Nonorganic milk comes from farms that are allowed to use GM cattle feed, routine antibiotic treatments and synthetic pesticides. These are not permitted on organic farms.'* Firstly, GM (Genetically Modified) feed is not allowed for organic cows in the Euoropean Union, but there is absolutely no evidence GM-fed cows give less healthy milk by virtue of eating GM feed. Secondly, as mentioned, antibiotics are also given to organic cows. Thirdly, there is no evidence of any significant difference in pesticide levels between organic and nonorganic milk (see *'Pesticides'* chapter for more information).

4. *'...organic farmers use traditional methods to produce purer, more natural organic milk that is good for you, the cows and the countryside.'* As explained in this book, organic milk is certainly not good for you, and it certainly is not good for the cows! Furthermore, organic milk (whether or not UHT) is worse for the countryside – it has a bigger impact on energy, environmental pollution,

and global warming compared to regular pasteurized milk.

The baseline that organic milk must '*come from cows that are not fed antibiotics and synthetic pesticides*' is loosely interpreted by just about all dairy farmers. Furthermore, the policing of such standards is practically non-existent in first world countries, let alone in less developed countries.

The Cancer-Causing Hormones Myth

Myth: Organic milk does not contain cancer-causing hormones.

Fact: Organic milk has as much cancer-causing hormones as nonorganic milk.

Virtually all dairy cows (including 'organic' dairy cows) are kept in a state of almost continuous pregnancy so as to maximize milk production. This continuous state of pregnancy produces milk rich in bovine growth hormones, known as 'Insulin-like Growth Factor 1' or IGF-1. No amount of organic diligence and no amount of pasteurization gets rid of these harmful IGF-1 hormones – they are a natural component of all dairy milk and cannot be removed. For the evidence see Appendix B.

Furthermore, IGF-1 survives human ingestion, so it is then absorbed into the body to cause harm. Many highly regarded studies show that IGF-1 in milk causes a multitude of diseases in humans.

Organic and nonorganic milk contain similar amounts of IGF-1. But UHT milk sends more of the IGF-1 into the body to cause harm (compared to regular pasteurized milk). For a fuller explanation see the chapter *The Lethal UHT Effect*.

In summary, organic milk is no different to regular pasteurized milk in terms of cancer-causing hormones. But organic UHT milk is worse because it gives the body a higher amount of IGF-1 hormones compared to regular pasteurized milk.

The Organic Milk Toxins Myth

Myth: Organic milk is free of harmful toxins.

Reality: Both organic and nonorganic milk have similar amounts of toxins.

Heavy metals such as lead, cadmium, zinc and mercury are highly toxic. Also, dioxins that result from incineration and smoke are extremely toxic. Heavy metals and dioxins, even in very small amounts, can accumulate in the human body and cause serious illnesses, including cancer.

How do these toxins enter into our bodies? The chain of events goes like this:

- Heavy metals and dioxins are created by industrial production processes and their emissions, road traffic fumes, smoke and dust, emissions of coal and gas-fired power stations, industrial waste and incineration, and many other environmental pollution activities, some man-made, and some natural such as forest fires and volcanic eruptions.

- These toxins enter the soil through the air, through water, through acid rain and weather patterns, and through actions that pollute the environment.

- The toxins then enter the food chain through plants. When we eat plants or when we consume milk from cows that eat plants, the toxins enter the human body.

So toxins enter the food chain through plants, fodder, hay, and anything that originally came from soil and water containing the toxins.[62] Virtually all pastures and arable farms contain toxins in varying degrees. Research shows that land near areas of heavy industry and industrial waste have higher concentrations of toxins in the soil compared to areas free of pollution, but nowhere escapes some degree of toxicity in the soil.

Heavy metals and dioxins are found in all kinds of dairy milk in varying degrees. Cows acquire toxins from the food they eat. The cow's body acts to accumulate and concentrate the toxins, and then pass them on through their milk.

Some heavy metals and dioxins mix with fertilizers, and *both organic and synthetic fertilizers* are at risk.[63] These toxins mostly come to us from the soil rather than from fertilizers, and hence into the grass and plants that grow in it. *Heavy metals and dioxins do not come from pesticides and chemicals used* in farming as these products are no longer manufactured with these toxins, and in any event strict laws prohibit the use of any farming products that contain such toxins.

Both organic cows and nonorganic cows are at equal risk of ingesting heavy metals and dioxins in the food and water they consume.

The amount of toxins found in milk will vary depending on farm locations, types of soil, etc. but 'organic farming' does not equate to a lower amount of heavy metals and dioxins. *Organic farming is meant to be about less pesticides, not less toxins.*

The dairy industry is quick to say that the level of heavy metals and dioxins in milk is well within safety limits set by regulatory bodies, and there is no danger to humans. But the truth is that any amounts of heavy metals and dioxins are harmful and there are no 'safe limits'. Furthermore, the amount of toxins in milk varies a great deal, and since milk is hardly ever tested for heavy metals and dioxins you simply don't know what cocktail of toxins you may be getting.

Of course, we also receive trace amounts of these toxins just by eating salads, vegetables and other plant foods, but these toxins are not concentrated as they are in milk. Consumed on a regular basis, dairy milk contributes more toxins to the human diet than any other food commodity, particularly UHT milk. This is so for two reasons:

1. Heavy metals and dioxins tend to be concentrated in the milk of any herbivore, including cows. These toxins are not destroyed by pasteurization or UHT.

2. Although levels of toxins are similar in organic and nonorganic milk, UHT milk gives you a higher proportion of toxins. For a fuller explanation please see chapter *The Lethal UHT Effect.*

- *Most dioxins come from industrial chlorination processes, incineration of municipal waste, and production of certain herbicides. The lipophilic nature of dioxins results in higher concentrations in the fat of animal and fish products, and their excretion via milk secretion in dairy cattle may result in relatively high concentrations of dioxin contamination in high-fat dairy products.*[67]

- Dioxins are highly toxic by-products of industrial processes. They penetrate the environment and the soil via air and water, and are then incorporated into food chains. The major source of human exposure (90% of the total) is the consumption of a wide variety of common foods (meat, fish and dairy products) containing small amounts of dioxins. Food contamination with dioxins leads to enhanced accumulation of these compounds in human tissues to the extent of exceeding acceptable level.[64]

- Dioxins are the most deadly substances ever assembled by man... 170,000 times more deadly than cyanide...[65]

- The level of dioxin in a single serving of the Ben & Jerry's World's Best Vanilla Ice Cream tested was almost 200 times greater than the "virtually safe [daily] dose" determined by the US Environmental Protection Agency.[66]

In conclusion, organic milk is no different to regular pasteurized milk in terms of toxins. But organic UHT milk is worse because it gives the body a higher amount of toxins compared to regular pasteurized milk. Also, there is a risk that people who buy organic milk are likely to consume more milk out of a false sense of security. By doing so they risk ingesting more toxins than otherwise.

'Organic consumers are more likely to consume more milk per day. Organic consumers are less sensitive to price effects.'[114]

The More Nutritious Myth

Myth: Organic milk is more nutritious than nonorganic milk.

Reality: Organic milk is not more nutritious than nonorganic milk.

We have mentioned that organic UHT milk is said to have a shelf life of up to 6 months, although typically the milk would be sold to consumers within a few weeks.

An extended expiration date enables organic dairies to ship their products farther and allows stores to receive shipments less often. *'Organic milk isn't produced in all parts of the country, so UHT is a way for companies to reach more customers.'*[29]

When milk is pasteurized this also greatly diminishes the nutrient content of the milk. Pasteurized milk has up to a 66 percent loss of vitamins A, D and E. Vitamin C loss usually exceeds 50 percent. Heat affects water soluble vitamins and can make them 38 percent to 80 percent less effective. Vitamins B6 and B12 are virtually destroyed during pasteurization.

Pasteurization also destroys beneficial enzymes, antibodies and lipase (an enzyme that breaks down fat). A lack of lipase impairs fat metabolism and the ability to properly absorb fat soluble vitamins A and D. (The dairy industry is aware of the diminished vitamin D content in commercial milk, so they fortify it with a form of this vitamin.)

As UHT milk is pasteurized to a much higher temperature, even more nutrients are destroyed compared to regular pasteurization. Some organic dairy farmers defend this by saying that UHT is necessary because many micro-organisms have become heat resistant and now survive ordinary pasteurization. (This makes you wonder whether it's safe to consume organic milk that is merely pasteurized!).

There is no escaping the fact that UHT renders organic milk virtually 'sterile', devoid of life-enhancing enzymes, sterols and healthy oils (and with few vitamins and minerals unless added later). This is why UHT milk is said to not require refrigeration until opened.

The FSA[61] (UK Foods Standards Agency) says organic milk does not offer any extra health benefits compared to conventional milk, and food watchdogs have rejected claims that expensive organic milk is any healthier than its conventional equivalent.

Equally, the USDA (US Department of Agriculture) says there is *'no conclusive evidence showing that organic food is more nutritious than conventionally grown food.'* And the USDA — even though it certifies organic food — doesn't claim that these products are safer or more nutritious.

Confusion arises because several studies around the world have found higher levels of nutrients in organic milk, particularly omega-3. Omega-3s are considered to cut consumers' risk of heart disease, and have been linked with better concentration in children and with better health generally.

A three-year study conducted at the Universities of Glasgow and Liverpool found organic milk contained 68 percent more omega-3 fatty acids on average than nonorganic milk.[158]

However, this study was carried in 2006 and since then other studies have not shown any significant difference in omega-3 between organic and nonorganic milk. Furthermore, the study was based on a group of carefully controlled cows given a rich diet of fresh pasture all the year round, a luxury that very few (if any) organic cows enjoy in commercial farming.

Also, the Glasgow study was based on raw milk, before it was pasteurized and homogenized. Milk processing has a drastic effect on omega-3 content. Indeed, if the intention is to inform the public, then any study into the nutritional content of milk will be largely invalidated unless based on the end product that is consumed.

The findings (of the Glasgow 2006 study) led 14 scientists from around the world to sign a letter asking the FSA[61] to recognise the nutritional advantages of organic milk.

Such a pronouncement would have been a huge boost to the standing of organic milk. However, the FSA has rejected any health benefits following consultations with leading experts.

A report published by the FSA accepts that organic milk *'can contain higher levels of types of fats called short-chain omega-3 fatty acids than conventionally produced milk'*. But it dismisses the significance of this, saying these are of 'limited health benefit' compared to the longer chain omega-3 fatty acids found in oily fish.

And, it adds: *'Therefore, organic milk consumed in volumes consistent with a healthy diet, would not provide sufficient amounts of long-chain omega-3 fatty acids to provide significant health benefits, over and above those associated with conventional milk.'*

The Chairman of the FSA, Dame Deirdre Hutton, confirmed the verdict in a letter to the academics behind the original study stating: *'It would therefore not be appropriate to advise consumers to switch to organic milk for reasons related to dietary health.'*

In another study (*Improving Sustainability in Organic and Low Input Food Production Systems'* carried out by Newcastle University and announced in March

2007)[60] it was reported that organic fruit and vegetables do indeed have a greater nutritional content than their nonorganic equivalents. Clearly, if you provide fruit and vegetables with a richer soil you are likely to end up with more nutritious produce, and the Newcastle project confirms this.

The project also found that organic milk was higher in amounts of omega-3 oils and antioxidants. To carry out the study the Newcastle project used a 725-acre farm attached to the University, and cows were allowed to graze freely (under carefully controlled conditions) on rich fresh organic pastures that included clover. *Raw* milk samples from organic and nonorganic cows were analyzed for the project. That is, no pasteurized or UHT milk was used in the project thus making the study somewhat irrelevant from the perspective of a milk consumer.

Clearly, if you feed cows a healthy, nutritious diet and keep them happy, the milk is going to be more nutritious than otherwise. Unfortunately, the vast majority of so-called organic cows do not have this kind of life, and consequently their milk is not significantly different to nonorganic cows.

This is confirmed by several studies showing that, at the very least, organic milk is not higher in vitamin content. For example, a University of Glasgow study carried in 2007 revealed that *'conventionally produced milk fat* [i.e. nonorganic milk] *had a higher mean content of vitamin A than organically produced milk fat, although there were no significant differences in the vitamin E or β-carotene contents between the two types of milk fat.*'[155]

Other research shows little difference in the nutritional value between organic and nonorganic milk. If anything, the nonorganic milk is shown to have a *higher* nutritional value when direct comparisons are made. For example, a Newcastle University study published in April 2008[160] found little nutritional difference between organic cows put to pasture (low input cows) and organic cows confined to sheds (high input cows).

But when low input organic and nonorganic cows were compared a significant difference was found. It was found that milk from nonorganic cows was significantly *higher* in antioxidants and conjugated linoleic acid. The study thought that perhaps the use of mineral NPK fertilisers in nonorganic pastures contributed to this.

The Newcastle study[160] also found that, as shown by other research, *'milk composition is known to change when switching from outdoor grazing to indoor forage-based diets in winter, however little is known about whether this dietary change affects the differential in milk quality between organic and [nonorganic milk]'.*

What is clear is that one cannot generalize about the nutritional value of organic milk vis-a-vis nonorganic milk since so many variables come into play.

The Newcastle study concluded that *'milk composition is affected by production systems, by mechanisms likely to be linked to the stage and length of the grazing period, and by diet composition, which will influence subsequent processing, sensory and potential qualities of the milk'.*

It is readily admitted that some other studies have shown organic milk to be marginally higher in nutritional content. Such studies have usually concentrated on a carefully controlled group of organic cows given a diet of fresh rich pastures.

A good example of this is a study often quoted by the milk industry, and carried out by a team from the Danish Institute of Agricultural Research in early 2005.[156]

The study concluded that *"Organically reared cows, which eat high levels of fresh grass, clover pasture and grass clover silage, produced milk which is on average 50% higher in Vitamin E (alpha tocopherol), 75% higher in beta carotene (which our bodies convert to Vitamin A) and two to three times higher in the antioxidants lutein and zeaxanthine than non-organic milk."*

Let's briefly look at this conclusion:

- Clearly, any cow fed an optimum diet of rich pastures in a stress-free environment is going to produce more nutritious milk. Unfortunately this does not apply to the vast majority of so-called organic cows.

- The study looked at raw milk only. The process of pasteurization nullifies to a large extent the amount of vitamin E. Up to 66% of vitamin E is lost through pasteurization, and even more through UHT. The trace amount of vitamin E that makes it to your glass of milk is too small to be of any consequence in terms of human health. Furthermore, vitamin E is available from a very wide variety of food sources (cereals, nuts, oils, grains, seeds, vegetables) and people generally are not short of vitamin E.

- The beta carotene content of milk is entirely dependent on a cow having a diet of pastures rich in beta carotene all the year round (plenty of fresh green grass and clover). As stated, most organic cows do not have such a diet. Although beta carotene is not destroyed by pasteurization temperatures, it is mostly destroyed by UHT temperatures.[157] Beta carotene converts to vitamin A in the human body, and this vitamin is widely available from animal produce, and from fruit and vegetables. It is generally not in short supply in the human diet, and vitamin A deficiency is rarely seen in developed countries.

- The Danish study stated that organic milk was *"two to three times higher in the antioxidants lutein and zeaxanthine than non-organic milk."* These are carotenoid pigments found in abundance in fruit and vegetables. Like beta carotene, lutein and zeaxanthine are entirely dependent on the cow's diet being high in fresh green grass and rich clover. There is no evidence that lutein and zeaxanthine are "two to three times higher" when *pasteurized* milk is compared. Furthermore, Lutein and zeaxanthine are almost totally destroyed by the high temperatures of UHT processing.

There is, of course, an easy way to test and compare the nutritional value of organic milk: simply take a *random* sample of different brands of organic milks and nonorganic milks from a variety of supermarket shelves. Do this over a period of time, putting the samples through rigorous laboratory analysis and compare the results. This would be a more valid and transparent comparison.

In fact this was done in a major University of Minnesota study in 2007/8 and the results clearly showed no nutritional difference between organic and nonorganic milk: *'Audited procedures found* [both types of milk] *to have the same nutrient content.'* [162]

In the USA this is what the American Institute for Cancer Research has to say: *'Demand for organic milk, which can sell for up to double the cost of other milk, is booming. Deciding whether to spend the extra money is not as clear-cut a decision as some suggest. People may turn to organic milk for health benefits, or environmental and animal rights' issues. But when evaluating the health claims, so far, research does not support a health advantage of organic over conventional milk for any segment of the population.*[30]

Although the nutritional content of milk depends on how the cow is fed, this is to a large extent rendered irrelevant by the high pasteurization temperatures that kill off most micro-organisms and damage many enzymes and other nutrients. Several studies have compared pasture-fed cows to cows fed hay and grain. British organic rules require that at least 60 per cent of a cow's feed over the course of a full year come from pastures or stored pasture-hay produced on the farm. This limits the amount of grain and feed rations the animals can consume.

Conventionally raised cows given a primarily pasture-based diet would have the same minor omega-3 levels as organic cows. In contrast to the UK, where the climate allows for pasture-based dairying for much of the year, the majority of organic milk in the US and Canada is from cows fed grain, soy and hay. Many conventional dairies in both these countries put their cows out to pasture when they can, and feed them indoors during the cold and dry months.

A number of research projects (mostly sponsored by the organic farming lobby) have highlighted apparent nutritional benefits in organic milk. Consequently, the FSA's findings that organic milk is no more nutritious than nonorganic milk have surprised and upset organic farming supporters as well as the scientists involved in the previously mentioned 2006 Glasgow and Liverpool study.

Here is the official view of the FSA [61] when it comes to answering the question: *Is organic milk more nutritious?*

'Whilst the nutrient profile of organic milk appears to be different from nonorganic milk, care must be taken when drawing conclusions as to the nutritional significance of this. Dairy sources of omega-3 polyunsaturated fatty acids are not a viable alternative to eating oily fish. Milk contains the shorter chain form of omega-3 polyunsaturated fatty acids (alpha-linolenic acid), while the forms present in oily fish are the long chain fatty acids (eicosapentaenoic (EPA) and docosahexaenoic acids (DHA)). Research has shown that the short chain form found in plant and dairy sources does not appear to be as beneficial as those found in oily fish, which have been shown to be protective for cardiovascular disease, and may also have beneficial effects on foetal development.'

As stated, it should be emphasized that the nutritional benefits attributable to organic milk mostly come from dairy cows allowed to graze freely on highly nutritious pastures for most of the year – such a small percentage of cows as to be insignificant. The image of free-range bovines frolicking in fields is just that – an image. What is meant to set apart the cows producing milk sold as organic is what they eat: grain that is not genetically modified and feed containing no animal by-products.

Many consumers assume that because organic farming requires that cows must have 'access to pasture' this means cows graze in fields most of the year. But current organic standards worldwide *do not require a specific length of time in pasture*. A cow can graze In pasture for only a very limited time and still produce milk that can then be certified organic.

The vast majority of organic cows (in the world generally) are confined to milk-producing sheds in the same way as nonorganic cows. A laboratory analysis of organic milk taken from such cows would reveal no significant nutritional difference compared to nonorganic milk.

But apart from the effect of cow feed on the nutritional value of UHT milk, a major consideration is the storage time of the milk. Studies show that the unrefrigerated storage of UHT cartons of milk (which can typically be for several months) greatly affects the nutrients in the milk.

Storage of UHT milk can significantly increase acidity and toxicity, and this in turn can affect how the vitamins and minerals are absorbed by the body when the milk is consumed – see *Appendix E: Effects of UHT Storage.*

We should remember that the long list of nutrients displayed on milk cartons is a list of nutrients that applied straight after pasteurization and homogenization, and **before** the milk was packaged and stored. It does not represent the nutrients in milk at the time of consumption (particularly in the case of UHT milk).

Some milk producers claim that organic milk is better for you because it contains omega-3 oil – this is a spurious claim for the following reasons:

Omega-3 levels in cows vary widely, both by season and between farms, including the organic ones. You really have no way of knowing if you're getting the higher omega-3 levels that the organic marketers seem to promise. Another factor is that milk simply isn't a major source of omega-3 in the human diet no matter how it is produced. A handful of nuts & seeds or a modest four ounce serving of salmon provides 60 to 90 times more omega-3s than an eight ounce glass of milk (organic or nonorganic). So called 'healthy' reduced-fat and low-fat milks have even less omega-3s because they are removed with the milk fat.

Furthermore, the nutritional value of omega-3 oil is largely destroyed at temperatures above 120ºF/49ºC. This is why all cold-pressed vegetable oils are made at temperatures below 120ºF/49ºC. When milk is pasteurized it is heated to a temperature of 162ºF/72ºC. And when milk is ultraheated it is heated to 285ºF/141ºC (and even higher in some UHT plants).

Clearly, you derive no benefit from any omega-3 oil in pasteurized or ultraheated milk (whether or not organic) because of the very high pasteurization temperatures.

Even if you were to consume *raw* (unpasteurized) milk of any kind you would only benefit from an insignificant amount of omega-3 in a pint of milk.

Omega-3 *fortified* dairy milk has been thoroughly evaluated by scientists who conclude that *'There is no firm evidence that adding omega-3 to milk improves a child's intelligence, and there is insufficient evidence to assert that omega-3 milk improves brain power.'*[31]

The idea that you should drink milk as a way of getting omega-3 oil is erroneous in the extreme. Apart from fish, omega-3 oils are available from a wide variety of food sources such as nuts, seeds, and plant oils (walnut, canola, olive, wheat germ, flax, soy, hemp and others). Omega-3 oil supplements in liquid form or as capsules are also widely available from retailers.

Some organic milk producers make a big song and dance about CLA (Conjugated Linoleic Acid). In fact there is no significant difference in CLA between organic and nonorganic milk: *'Organic milk has a higher proportion of polyunsaturated to monunsaturated fatty acids and of n-3 fatty acids than conventional milk. There was no difference between organic and conventional milk with respect to the proportion of CLA or vaccenic acid.'*[1]

It has been suggested that organic cows fed on pasture rather than grain have higher levels of CLA, but there is no evidence for this. Michael Pariza, professor of food microbiology and toxicology at the University of Wisconsin, and a leading expert on linoleic acid in dairy products, says grass feeding by itself does not assure increased CLA. He and Bauman (a professional colleague) both note that cows fed mixed grains with soybeans or other additions can produce milk that has higher CLA levels than milk from grass-fed cows.

In another study already mentioned (Glasgow & Liverpool Study, 2006[158]), and much quoted by the milk industry, it was concluded that there was no significant difference in CLA between organic and nonorganic cows. This in spite of the fact that the study was based on organic cows fed a rich fresh pasture all the year round.

The amount of CLA in one hundred grams of milk (raw or pasteurized) is a miniscule amount, just 0.46-

1.78g.[100] To acquire any significant amount of CLA from milk you would have to consume thousands of grams of milk fat!

CLAs are made up of exactly the same components as regular linoleic acid, just in a different molecular arrangement. CLA is classified as a trans fatty acid, and Linoleic acid is an omega-6 polyunsaturated fat.

Linoleic acid is available from a wide variety of food sources such as margarine, dairy products, vegetables oils, and many vegetables and processed foods. It is usually not in short supply in the diet – we generally receive too much omega 6 in the diet and not enough omega 3.

There has been much excitement about CLA because some studies have shown that CLA can help get rid of surplus body fat and prevent disease. Even if CLA proves to help with weight loss, given the small amount in milk, this would be far outweighed by the weight gain caused by milk fat!

Virtually all CLA studies on weight loss, cancer, cardiovascular disease, insulin sensitivity, diabetes and immune function have been conducted on *animals* and it has been acknowledged that variations exist between different animals' responses to CLAs. A 2006 review of 17 studies on humans concluded that CLA does not affect body weight or body composition and has a limited effect on immune function.[145]

Some detrimental effects of CLA have been observed in mice and some reports suggest that CLAs can increase the risk of cancer[146] and other diseases:

CLA may increase the risk of heart disease for overweight subjects. In a study, overweight volunteers who took 4.5 grams of Conjugated linoleic acid (CLA) daily for one year had an increase in their blood levels of lipoprotein(a), a risk factor for heart disease.[148]

CLA may increase risk of diabetes. Several studies indicate that the use of CLA by overweight people may increase insulin resistance, possibly increasing the risk of developing diabetes.[147] However, this evidence is controversial, and other studies report no changes in insulin sensitivity.

CLA may increase the risk of liver steatosis (fatty liver) by reducing leptin and adiponectin, and then increasing secretion of insulin and hepativc lipid content. These observations cast doubt on the safety of dietary supplements containing CLA.[149]

The reported side effects of taking CLA supplements include diarrhoea, bloating, flatulence, and stomach upset.

The dairy industry sees CLA as a marketing opportunity and research into producing CLA-enriched milk by manipulating the diet of dairy cows is well underway.

Given the current knowledge on CLA, there does not seem to be any benefit in consuming milk with CLA, and it should certainly not be a reason for choosing organic milk.

The Antibiotics Myth

Myth: Organic milk contains less or no antibiotics compared to nonorganic milk.

Fact: When it comes to antibiotics there is no difference between organic and nonorganic milk.

Nonorganic cows are often given antibiotics as a matter of course. But most people do not realize that organic cows are also often given antibiotics. Thus, even though organic milk is not meant to contain antibiotics, it does.

How is this so? Organic farming stipulates that no antibiotics are to be used unless needed for the medical treatment of an animal. Furthermore, most organic standards allow limited use of antibiotics.[2]

What happens in practice is that antibiotics are given to organic cows whenever illness is detected. Dairy farmers know that if they do not do this the cows become diseased and less productive.

In some countries, such a the USA, once an organic cow is given antibiotics, it should never be used again for milking. As a consequence, when organic cows fall ill they are often left untreated so that milking can continue until the cow is too ill to produce milk. It is also known that some organic farmers will reintroduce a treated cow into milk production when it has recovered rather than lose thousands of dollars invested in the cow.[162]

Clearly, many organic cows are not given antibiotics *routinely* in the way that nonorganic cows are treated. Nevertheless, any animal that is forced into a state of permanent pregnancy and lactation (and little exercise) is going to be more susceptible to illness. Just like nonorganic cows, organic cows are forced into becoming milk-producing machines, and hence need just as many antibiotics.

There is no rule that says antibiotics cannot be given to an organic cow if required on 'medical grounds'. If a farmer decides that a cow in an organic herd needs to be treated with antibiotics, she is not meant to be returned to the herd for a set period (typically 12 months according to organic farming rules in some countries such as the UK). In practice, no farmer can allow a 'healthy' cow to have a one-year vacation from milk production! For a dairy farmer this is a complete farce because in practice no milk producer can afford to keep cows idle for a year just because they've been given an antibiotic. On that basis virtually the whole organic herd would be out of action!

In nonorganic herds, milk from cows that receive antibiotics is not meant to be used until tests show the milk is antibiotic-free. So neither organic or nonorganic cows are meant to be used in milk production unless clear of antibiotics. In practice, this never happens, otherwise almost all dairy cows would be taken out of milk production.

To resolve this, tanks of raw milk are routinely tested to control antibiotic content. Such 'spot tests' give a kind of traffic light YES/NO answer and have a built-in margin of error. If antibiotics above a certain level are detected, the milk from that particular batch is discarded or used for cheese-making and other dairy products. Trace amounts of antibiotics are allowed, otherwise no milk (whether organic or not) would ever reach supermarket shelves.

'It is doubtful whether antibiotics get into non-organic milk. It's illegal to give antibiotics to a lactating cow. Farmers are responsible for any antibiotics that show up in tanker-truck samples, which would force the dumping of the entire truck's contents.' (Stephanie Hill, dairy specialist and assistant professor of animal science at North Carolina Agricultural & Technical State University in Greensboro, USA).

'A 2007/8 study looked at more than 200 samples of regular pasteurized milk and organic milk from retail stores across the U.S.A. Audited procedures found [both types of milk] *to have the same nutrient content. None contained antibiotics.'*[162]

Generally, milk testing is self-regulated throughout the world. Here is a brief description of how this works:

The milk processing companies themselves carry out the testing. Typically, a sample is taken from the milk just before it is loaded into a milk tanker. This is done every time a milk tanker goes to a dairy farm to collect milk.

The milk samples are collected by dairy companies and stored for a week or so before being discarded. But before being discarded one or two samples are chosen at random for testing. If any samples fail the testing the dairy farmer is penalized by receiving a much lower price for that particular batch of milk. This method ensures that dairy farmers are kept on their guard as they never know when their particular milk may be tested.

In general then, only a small fraction of the milk that reaches the consumer is actually tested for antibiotics. This applies to both organic and nonorganic milk since no distinction is made between the two in terms of sampling and testing procedures.

It should be mentioned that most countries in the world have government agencies that also do testing for antibiotics in milk. This acts as a kind of back-up to the testing carried out by the milk industry itself. But such testing is done on a very small 'token' scale. For example in the United Kingdom, DEFRA does random milk testing on about 0.12% of the milk produced (that's about one test per 15,000 tons of milk in a UK market that produces about 12 millions tons of milk per year).

All milk then, whether organic or nonorganic, contains antibiotics in varying degrees, with little or no difference between the two. The author makes the following challenge: *take any random sample of organic and nonorganic milk from various brands on supermarket shelves – do this over a period of time. Put the samples through rigorous scientific laboratory analysis for traces of antibiotics. Compare organic and nonorganic milk. There is unlikely to be any significant difference between the two types of milk.*

Dairy milk contains traces of a variety of antibiotics, one of these being penicillin. Such antibiotics are bad for humans because they weaken the immune system and make you more prone to disease by creating resistance in the body's bacteria.

This happens because the continual exposure to small levels of antibiotics in milk causes a modification of "good" bacteria in the intestine leading to vitamin and mineral deficiencies and a greater tendency to contract infections.

This also leads to drug-resistant strains of bacteria inside your body, making you less capable of responding to medication. Furthermore, the trace amounts of penicillin that are found in most pasteurized milk can be hazardous to people allergic to penicillin.

In the book *Killers Within*[3] the authors explain why antibiotics continue to be given in such high quantities to farm animals such as chickens, pigs, and cows: *"...the reason is that antibiotics are in fact powerful growth promoters. This explains why dairy cows are usually so overdosed with antibiotics."*

Dr. Neil Barnard (The Physicians Committee for Responsible Medicine, USA) says:

'Milk is extracted from cows that are kept producing milk with the help of hormones, long after they need it for their calves. The cows are fed commercially created feeds that may include hay, grain,

*cardboard, and wood shavings. They are regularly plied with large amounts of **antibiotics** to treat or fend off infections, which then find their way into the milk.*

To summarize, it may be argued that organic milk contains less antibiotics than nonorganic milk, but this would be a false argument. In fact, although organic cows may receive less antibiotics than nonorganic cows, both types of milk will end up with similar trace amounts of antibiotics. This is so because the antibiotic testing procedure for both types of milk is the same. This is the case in Europe and America, and is likely to be the same in other parts of the world. *There is no separate antibiotic testing procedure for organic cows.*

It may also be argued that the 'small, trace amounts of antibiotics' are not enough to affect health. This is not so – many studies show that the daily ingestion of trace amounts of antibiotics are the principal reason for increased illness arising from weakened immunity. Antibiotic resistance in humans is a major health issue in the world today – it is caused by the drip-feed ingestion of low-level antibiotics in the diet, not by occasional medication prescribed by a physician.

The Cow Treatment Myth

Myth: Organic cows are treated better than nonorganic cows.

Reality: Most organic cows suffer more, and are subject to the same harsh treatment given to nonorganic cows.

It is said that organic dairy farming can cause less suffering to dairy cows than conventional dairy farming. In some "show case" instances this may be the case; nevertheless, the conditions for most dairy cows are far from ideal, with many animals often suffering from diseases such as mastitis and lameness.

A six month study of the major animal health and welfare constraints in *organic* livestock systems was completed by The Department of Agriculture at the University of Reading, United Kingdom, by the Veterinary Epidemiology and Economics Research Unit (VEERU). Thirty four dairy farms were surveyed. The highest ranking disease problem in organic cows was mastitis. Infertility, milk fever and lameness were also commonly perceived problems.[134]

In order to lactate, all cows need to be made pregnant. In organic and nonorganic herds, male calves are a by-product and are usually taken away from their mothers within 24 hours to be slaughtered or raised for beef. There is no such thing as 'humane 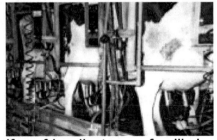 milk' - the only truly welfare-friendly type of milk is non-dairy and obtained from plants.

Another myth is that organic cows are allowed to roam free on pesticide-free pastures. Nothing could be further from the truth. The rules laid down for organic farming say nothing about giving cows space to roam free. The vast majority of organic cows are kept in the same kind of conditions as nonorganic cows, often confined to small spaces.

Stephanie Hill, a dairy specialist and assistant professor of animal science at North Carolina

Agricultural & Technical State University in Greensboro, USA, says:

'The image of smiley, happy cows on organic farms is not true to life. Since organic producers can't use conventional methods of treating illness, organic dairy farming makes it likelier that a sick cow will be culled, either by being cut from the herd or killed outright. And today's land constraints make it difficult to adhere to the access-to-pasture rule.'

With consumer demand for organic products continuing to grow, more large corporations are entering the organic market. To maximize profits, some of these companies don't follow organic standards but still label products as organic. For example, Horizon Organic and Aurora Organic, sold by Wal-Mart and other retailers in the USA, continue to produce "organic" milk under factory-farm conditions that few reasonable people would consider truly organic.

According to the US *Organic Consumers Association*, half of Horizon's "organic" milk today comes from what can only be considered "factory" dairy feedlots – as does much of Aurora's organic milk.

This is what Ronnie Cummins of the *Organic Consumers Association* has to say on the matter:

'Rather than buy organic calves that have been raised from birth on organic farms, these companies seem to have discovered that it's cheaper to buy conventional calves that have been raised on conventional farms, install them in factory feedlots, then milk them and call it organic.'

The situation has become so alarming that the US Organic Consumers Association ultimately called for a boycott, and many knowledgeable consumers are now avoiding the Horizon brand entirely.

Dean Foods has pushed for lower organic standards in the United States and to allow industrial-style production to be called "organic."

Do not imagine that organic cows are treated any better than nonorganic cows. *'There are certain dairies where 10 months out of the year the organic cows are confined and fed out of a trough, and then two months of the year when they're just about to give birth they're in the pasture,'* says Jim Riddle, who chairs the US *National Organic Standards Board.*

Kim Severson (an award winning food writer and author) wrote in the New York Times (*An Organic Cash Cow*, November 9, 2005) that:

"The ethos of organic milk… that it comes from a cow which had "access to pasture", is a term so vague it could mean that a cow might spend most of its milk-producing life confined to a feed lot eating grain and not grass."

No doubt some dairy farmers do indeed give their organic cows a better life compared to nonorganic cows, but such farming methods will always remain in the minority by virtue of being deemed to be commercially nonviable. Furthermore, just because a dairy cow is 'treated more humanely' it does not follow that therefore the milk is better for your health.

One thing is clear, the vast majority of so-called organic cows go through a life of greater suffering and disease compared to nonorganic cows. This is so because organic cows are not properly medicated when they become ill.

- *Organic cow's milk is loaded with as much saturated fat and cholesterol as regular milk, and it is often contaminated with pus and blood from cows who had udder infections and weren't given medicine because, if they were, the farmers wouldn't be able to label their milk organic. The dairy herd is sick— these are sick and diseased cows, producing pus-filled milk that even industry standards call 'unhealthy.'* [126]

- Dr. Chuck Guard, professor of veterinary medicine at Cornell University, has stated that it pains him that many technological advancements in animal medicine are prohibited for use on organic farms. He explains how organic farms don't use drugs to control parasites, worms, infections and illness in their herds: *"Drugs take away pain and suffering. Proponents of organic food production have thrown away these medical tools, and the result is unnecessary pain and suffering for the animals."*

- *If a cow on an organic dairy needs to be treated for a bacterial disease (infection in her udder, infection in her uterus after calving, pneumonia, etc.), the organic rules* [in the USA] *say she must be treated and that she can <u>never</u> again be used to produce organic milk. A new dairy cow costs about $2,000. Treating her properly when she is sick on an organic dairy is a major loss. The truth is that some sick cows on organic dairies are left to fend for themselves without treatment….Sick cows on organic dairies may be treated with unproven, untested, and questionably effective products with unknown effects on the milk the cow produces. You have to ask yourself just how humane it is to withhold medically proven therapy from a sick cow so that you can continue to sell higher-priced milk to the organic market.* [162]

The Environment Myth

Myth: Organic milk is better for the environment.

Reality: Organic milk causes more harm to the environment compared to nonorganic milk.

It is well known in the farming industry that organic milk – pint for pint – is less energy efficient (compared to nonorganic milk) because it does not use many of the chemicals created specifically to increase milk production.

Organic milk production may have that "hippy" feel of loving animals and the earth, but organic milk is primarily about the quality of food you put into your body, not the amount of land it took to make milk, or the energy it took to deliver the milk to your refrigerator.

Another factor is that most *organic* milk in the world comes from small farms, whereas as most *nonorganic* milk comes from vast milk-producing 'farms/factories' that house hundreds of cows. Economies of scale mean that the supply chain for organic milk has a far greater impact on the environment, pint-for-pint, compared to nonorganic milk. Collecting, storing, and distributing organic milk from lots of small farms takes up far more energy, transportation, etc. than nonorganic milk with its large-scale well-established infrastructure.

In a project titled '*Improving Sustainability in Organic and Low Input Food Production Systems*' carried out by Newcastle University (UK) and announced in March 2007[60] it was reported that '*energy use and green house gas emissions per hectare on organic farms are lower than on conventional farms, particularly in dairy farming. Energy use and green house gas emissions per Mg of milk in organic dairy farming are about 80% and 90% respectively of that in conventional dairy farming.'*

This project was based on a study of cows in carefully controlled conditions. Also, as the study readily admits, variations were found in environmental impact when results from farms in other countries were analyzed. Furthermore, in assessing the environmental impact, supply chain issues were not considered. Although not the intention of the study, clearly, any investigation into the environmental impact of milk must fully take into account supply chain issues.

A comprehensive 200-page study carried out by DEFRA[4], concluded that *'while many organic products had lower ecological impacts than conventional methods using fertilisers and pesticides, this is counterbalanced by other organic foods - such as __milk__, tomatoes and chicken - which are significantly less energy efficient and can be more polluting than intensively-farmed equivalents.'*

Further evidence comes from the book 'How to Live a Low-Carbon Life':

'Organic dairy cows are worse for the climate. They produce less milk so their methane emissions per litre of milk are higher.' [113]

Evidence that organic milk production is not less polluting or less harmful to the environment (compared to nonorganic milk) comes from the following fact: intensive dairy farming generally has a lower impact on the environment, pint for pint, compared to organic dairy farming.

All types of dairy farming produce polluting discharges and have an effect on the environment. But to suggest that intensive dairy farming produces more pollution and has a bigger effect on the environment is not in accordance with the research in this subject.

'It is incorrect to suggest that [greater pollution and a greater impact on the environment] *is due to more intensive farming methods. In other words, it is the production of more milk that has increased environmental pollution and not the intensification of production. The higher input farm* [nonorganic milk] *produces significantly more milk per hectare (75%). However, the effect on…the environment is similar to the organic farm. High input systems, when managed well, allow greater production of milk-solids per hectare, thereby helping to maintain natural ecosystems, while not having additional adverse effects on the environment.'*[161]

In other studies it is clear that when the full supply-chain is taken into account organic milk has a significantly greater impact in terms of energy use and greenhouse gas emissions. This is because, as mentioned, most organic farming is small scale and uses more energy (transportation, storage, etc) to transport the organic milk to the consumer's table. Nonorganic milk, with its well established supply chains, economies of scale and minimum storage times, is more likely to have a lower environmental impact, pint for pint.

But even though nonorganic milk production and distribution has a lower impact on the environment (pint for pint), it does not mean that keeping cows in sheds all their lives is better than putting them out to pasture. Keeping any kind of animal locked up for life in artificial circumstances is totally wrong, and for this reason alone all types of dairy milk should be avoided.

Clearly, if you must buy milk it is better to obtain it from sources that do allow cows to pasture, regardless of quality, price, or environmental impact. But sadly, most organic cows are kept locked up just about as much as nonorganic cows.

No doubt there will be exceptions. There will be farms that produce organic milk and sell it locally, with a small supply-chain that has little impact on the environment. But taken as a whole, organic milk, pint for pint, has a considerably bigger impact on the environment (compared to regular pasteurized milk) when economies of scale and all the factors in the supply-chain are taken into account.

Thousand Year Milk Myth

This myth is not specific to organic milk but it is included for the sake of completeness. The milk industry generally defends the consumption of milk by saying the following:

'Milk has been part of the human diet for thousands of years. Despite the fact that milk is one of the most nutritionally complete foods available, there are many myths relating to its consumption that blame milk and dairy foods for a variety of ailments. Many of these myths have been part of the folklore for centuries and are not founded on science.'

Let's briefly analyse this statement. There is absolutely no evidence that dairy milk has been consumed by humans on any kind of regular basis for 'thousands of years'. Archaeologists have discovered that as far back as 6000 BC cheese had been made from cow's and goat's milk and stored in tall jars. Egyptian tomb murals of 2000 BC show butter and cheese being made. Other murals, which show milk being stored in skin bags suspended from poles, show a knowledge of dairy husbandry at that time.

But these fragments of history do not mean that the human race has been consuming milk on a regular daily basis for thousands of years. Furthermore, even if a few 'privileged' people were consuming milk thousands of years ago, it would have been sporadic, and it would have been raw, organic milk free of disease and pollution (bearing no resemblance to modern-day pasteurized milk). The amount consumed would have been very little, as milk would only have been available when cows happened to be lactating.

The regular mass consumption of milk only started about two hundred years ago when milk processing and distribution became possible with scientific advances.

However, whatever the kind of milk (raw, organic, pasteurized or UHT) it does not mean that cow's milk is healthy for humans to consume. Just because a product has been consumed for hundreds or even thousands of years, it does not follow that the product must be healthy and nutritious. Many things that were consumed by our remote ancestors were not healthy but they were consumed as a matter of survival (eat or die of hunger). Clearly, it is better to consume dairy milk if the *only* alternative is starvation and death, but it does not follow that dairy milk is therefore good for you.

The dairy industry often promotes milk by saying that it is *'one of the most nutritionally complete foods available.'* Naturally, dairy milk is very much a 'complete food' for a baby calf. Human milk is a complete food for a baby human. But it does not follow that dairy milk is a 'complete food' for human children and adults. This is false logic carried to extreme.

Which milk is worst?

All kinds of dairy milk are bad for health without exception. Furthermore, all kinds of organic milk are worse for health (compared to nonorganic milk) for a variety of reasons as explained in this book.

Clearly, UHT or long life milk is the worst kind of milk to consume, whether or not organic. As already explained, the combination of UHT homogenization & pasteurization serve to greatly increase the amount of harmful cow hormones (and other substances) that enter the human body. This in turn increases illness and the risk of various types of cancer.

So UHT organic and UHT nonorganic milks are the worst choices for health. Do not fall into the trap of thinking that UHT organic milk may be marginally lower in antibiotics and pesticides – there is no evidence for this.

In any event, consumers who buy organic milk in the belief that is has lower antibiotics and pesticides are likely to consume a greater amount out of a false sense of security.

For such consumers, a higher consumption of organic milk may result in poorer health from all the other bad aspects of milk: obesity, clogged respiratory system, cataracts, cancer, diabetes, brain disease, and so on.

When it comes to choosing between *non-UHT* organic and *non-UHT* regular milk, the choice is clear: non-UHT organic milk is unhealthier because it is more likely to have a higher pus count and because it is more likely to contain harmful viruses and bacteria that cause disease (see chapters titled 'Pus' and 'Disease'). Additionally, organic milk production causes greater suffering for most organic cows, and is worse for the environment and global warming (see chapters titled "Cow Treatment Myth' and 'Environment Myth').

To summarize, if you absolutely must consume dairy milk, clearly it is best to avoid all kinds of UHT/long life milk, whether or not organic. This cannot be over-emphasized: *avoid UHT*. If choosing between *non-UHT organic* and *non-UHT regular milk*, you will know from reading this book that it is best to go for non-UHT regular milk.

The following table gives an at-a-glance comparison of which milk is worst – see next page.

Which Milk is Worst?

This is not a list of all aspects of dairy milk.
It is a list of just some aspects to consider when comparing organic and nonorganic milk.

1 tick: item applies (see KEY below this table).
2 ticks: worse than 1 tick (unhealthier or worse).

Item (see KEY below table)	Regular pasteurized	Organic pasteurized	Organic UHT
A. Storage	Not applicable	Not applicable	✓✓
B. Cancer	✓	✓	✓✓
C. Nutrition	✓	✓	✓✓
D. Fats	✓	✓	✓✓
E. Acidity	✓	✓	✓✓
F. Sex Hormones	✓	✓	✓✓
G. Toxins	✓	✓	✓✓
H. Calcification	✓	✓	✓✓
I. Osteoporosis	✓	✓	✓✓
J. Disease	✓	✓✓	✓✓
K. Pus	✓	✓✓	✓✓
L. Price	✓	✓✓	✓✓
M. Environment	✓	✓✓	✓✓
N. Cruelty	✓	✓✓	✓✓
O. Consumption	✓	✓✓	✓✓

KEY:

The comments that follow refer to the above table and summarize some of the issues examined throughout this book.

Key: A. Storage. The storage of UHT milk for several weeks or months before consumption has a dramatic and detrimental effect on the quality and nutritional value of the milk. See Appendix E.

Key: B. Cancer. All dairy milk contains IGF-1, a cancer-causing hormone. Organic UHT milk gives you more IGF-1 than regular pasteurized milk for the reasons explained in this book (see chapter *The Lethal UHT Effect*).

Key: C. Nutrition. Dairy milk provides little in the way of nutrition because pasteurization kills most enzymes, vitamins, and omega oils. Also, many minerals are not absorbed because they stick to milk casein and are flushed from the body. Organic UHT milk provides even less nutrition because of ultraheating which destroys more nutrients.

Key: D. Fats. Dairy milk provides harmful fats. Organic UHT provides more harmful fat because UHT creates more trans-fats.

Key: E. Acidity. Dairy milk causes high acidity when consumed; this is bad for health. UHT milk is more acidic because of storage (Appendix E) and because the higher pasteurization temperatures of UHT make the protein in milk more acidic.

Key: F. Sex Hormones. All dairy milk contains bovine sex hormones which increase the risk of cancer and other illnesses. With UHT, a greater proportion of sex hormones make it into the blood stream. For a full explanation see chapter *The Lethal UHT Effect*.

Key: G. Toxins. All dairy milk contains harmful toxins in varying degrees. These come from the environment (from the soil into pastures, from acid rain, from water, and from polluted air). Cows ingest toxins from the environment, regardless of the organic or nonorganic food they eat. These toxins (heavy metals and dioxins) are then concentrated in the cows milk. With UHT, a greater proportion of toxins (see chapter *The Lethal UHT Effect)* make it into the blood stream. The toxins can then be taken to many parts of the body to cause harm.

Key: H. Calcification. Organic UHT is more likely to cause harmful calcification compared to regular pasteurized milk. This is so because the higher acidity of UHT has the effect of increasing the amount of calcium that is dumped by the bloodstream in all parts of the body to cause many serious diseases. (More information: www.milkimperative.com).

Key: I. Osteoporosis. Organic UHT is more likely to increase the risk of osteoporosis compared to regular pasteurized milk. This is so because the higher acidity of UHT has the effect of eroding a greater amount of bone-making cells. (More information: www.milkimperative.com).

Key: J. Disease. Dairy milk promotes a variety of diseases because of toxins, hormones, mucus-forming casein, and other harmful substances. Consider the following two points:

1. *Organic milk* farming employs methods that greatly increase the amount of pathogens. Farmyard animal waste and sludge is commonly used as fertilizer but some of the pathogens in the waste material are not broken down by earthworms and insects. This significantly increases the amount of pathogens that come into contact with cows, causing contamination and illness in cows, and even in milk consumers.

> 'Some kinds of bacteria in dairy milk are able to survive pasteurization, causing Johne's Disease, Crohns Disease, and IBS...'[6]

> "Organic farms don't use drugs to control parasites, worms, infections and illness in their herds. Drugs take away pain and suffering. Proponents of organic food production have thrown away these medical tools, and the result is unnecessary pain and suffering for the cows." (Dr. Chuck Guard, professor of veterinary medicine at Cornell University).

2. Organic UHT milk promotes more disease than regular pasteurized milk because of UHT milk processing: more casein, toxins, damaged whey proteins, galactose, and other disease-promoting substances enter the bloodstream (see chapter The Lethal UHT Effect).

Key: K. Pus. All dairy milk contains pus. Research shows that organic milk is likely to contain more pus because of restrictions in the use of antibiotics.

Key: L. Price. Why pay extra money? Organic milk costs 50% to 100% more, yet offers no additional health benefits (and is worse for your health!) compared to regular pasteurized milk.

Key: M. Environment. Organic milk is worse for the environment, both in terms of energy use and green house gas emissions. This is so because organic milk uses more energy in the supply chain compared to regular pasteurized milk.

Also, organic cows produce more methane which is bad for the environment:

'Organic dairy cows are worse for the climate. They produce less milk so their methane emissions per litre of milk are higher.' [113]

Key: N. Cruelty. Organic farming causes more cruelty to cows compared to conventional dairy farming. For full details please see *"The Cow Treatment Myth"* in this book. Here is a brief summary:

Organic cows are kept in the same kind of conditions as nonorganic cows, often confined to small spaces. Most suffer from the same diseases as nonorganic cows, such as mastitis and lameness. Only a tiny number of showcase organic farms treat their cows well (usually sponsored by organic farming interests).

To maximize profits, some milk companies don't follow organic standards but still label products as organic. For example, Horizon Organic and Aurora Organic, sold by Wal-Mart and other retailers in the USA continue to produce "organic" milk under factory-farm conditions that few reasonable people would consider truly organic.

'There are certain dairies where 10 months out of the year the organic cows are confined and fed out of a trough, and then two months of the year when they're just about to give birth they're in the pasture,' says Jim Riddle, who chairs the US National Organic Standards Board.

No doubt some dairy farmers do indeed give their organic cows a better life compared to nonorganic cows, but such farming methods will always remain in the minority by virtue of being deemed to be commercially nonviable.

Dr. Chuck Guard, professor of veterinary medicine at Cornell University, has stated that it pains him that many technological advancements in animal medicine are prohibited for use on organic farms. He explains how organic farms don't use drugs to control parasites, worms, infections and illness in their herds: *"Drugs take away pain and suffering. Proponents of organic food production have thrown away these medical tools, and the result is unnecessary pain and suffering for the animals."*

Key: O. Consumption. Given that all kinds of dairy milk are bad for health, organic milk is the worst in the sense that you are likely to consume more than otherwise. Milk consumers do this out of a false sense of security. Market research shows that organic milk consumers buy more milk than otherwise by virtue of it being organic – they buy it and consume more out of a feeling that *'if it's organic it must be good'*. Some people even say they would not buy dairy milk at all unless it was organic!

***

Clearly, the best choice of all is to avoid all kinds of dairy milk, and switch to non-dairy milk.

Switching to non-dairy milk is easy as supermarkets and health food stores now sell a variety of milks made from soy, rice, oats, almonds and other varieties. Also, it's easy to make non-dairy milk at home. For information about recipes on how to make delicious non-dairy milk go to: www.about-milk.info.

Epilogue: Picture of seduction

When you enter a supermarket you enter a carefully choreographed world where *every last detail* is planned to entice shoppers to spend money. As you approach the refrigerated section that contains dairy milk you see a big selection of dairy milk cartons, all professionally packaged and arranged for maximum appeal. The long rows of colourful milk cartons project an air of fresh coolness and reassurance which plays on the unconscious mind.

As you gaze for a few moments at the rows of milk cartons carefully displayed to attract maximum custom (see picture), you occasionally see people taking a milk carton from the good-looking display. The people buying milk are a mix of nice ordinary people: a family, a housewife, a vicar, a teenager, and a

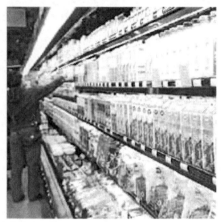

business man. You think: *Can so many people not know the truth about milk?* You look closely at a few cartons and you see a cornucopia of health-promoting messages: *lactose free, low fat, natural, organic, healthy, good for bones, etc.*

You pick out a carton of organic milk and see a nice picture of happy cows grazing in lush green pastures. Words like *pure, omega-3, calcium, no pesticides, no antibiotics, environment friendly farming*, etc. Jump out. You also see several official-looking organic certifications and guarantees of quality, giving a strong impression of credibility and authority.

You unconsciously make an association between these health-promoting messages, the credibility, the cool enticing display of milk cartons, and the people buying milk (*'they cannot all be wrong about milk'*). Deep down in your mind you think to yourself: *If dairy milk were truly bad for health supermarkets wouldn't be allowed to sell it! Anyhow, I use so little it won't make any difference.'* This picture of seduction is reinforced by television, magazine, billboard and other advertising seen by you in recent days promoting dairy milk. You buy the milk.

Different versions of this *picture of seduction* are played out daily, millions of times all over the world. Many people have vaguely heard that milk may be fattening or that it causes lactose intolerance, but it does not stop them being seduced into buying yet more milk. The message to take on board is simple: don't be seduced!

***

Appendix A: Super Harmful Casein

Casein is bad news for two reasons:

1. Casein causes illness: it promotes mucus congestion, inviting disease and preventing the immune system from keeping harmful viruses and bacteria at bay.

2. Casein helps micronized fat globules carry harmful substances from the milk right into the small intestine where they are more likely to be digested and absorbed into the body and the bloodstream.

Casein molecules are sticky and when milk is homogenized and pasteurized, the casein coats the newly micronized fat globules and 'seals in' the harmful substances that are bound with the fat globules.

This helps in the efficient digestion of the fat globules and the transfer of the globules' cargo (damaged whey proteins, heavy metals, IGF-1 hormones, other toxins) across the intestine wall and into the body.

Without casein, most of the harmful substances would be excreted rather than be absorbed into the body.

- *There is insufficient* [fat globule] *membrane to coat the newly formed surface completely, consequently the globules in homogenized milk are coated by a membrane which mostly consists of casein, with some whey protein.* [123]

- *The sudden increase in globule numbers causes a proportional increase in their surface area, which the original globule membranes are insufficient to cover. The naked fat surface attracts casein particles, which stick and create an artificial coat (nearly a third of the milk's casein ends up on the globules). The casein particles both weigh the fat globules down and interfere with their usual clumping: and so the fat remains evenly dispersed in the milk.*[124]

- *The ultra-high-pressure homogenization (UHPH) was found to increase the amount of non-sedimentable caseins (κ, α_{as1} and α_{as2}) in the serum [blood]. Electron microscopy showed formation of smaller [casein] particles...It was concluded that UHPH was capable of modifying the structural properties of casein micelles.*[141]

Casein is highly acidic with a pH rating of 4.6. During digestion, a significant amount of casein amino acids are not digested and end up as acidic wastes. When acidic wastes occur in the intestines, this can have four detrimental effects on the body: [143]

1. Appetite cravings are more likely or more pronounced (toxic acidic food residues create abnormal hunger pangs).

2. Acidic wastes encourage the body to store more surplus body fat.

3. Acidic wastes make for a less alkaline environment in the body. This in turn reduces the production of food-digesting enzymes. The more enzymes that break down food molecules in the gastrointestinal tract, the less food remains undigested. Over time, undigested food in the intestines cause health problems such as obesity and cancer.

4. Acidic wastes rob the body of nutrients. As the acidic wastes leave the body the wastes become

stuck to minerals which would otherwise be digested.

For the technically minded, note that casein itself is not absorbed when milk is consumed. Casein is broken down by the digestion process, and then casein amino acids are absorbed through the intestine wall into the body. Some of these amino acids have *"opioid properties which can potentially affect the body in a variety of ways including suppression of the immune system."*[142]

This is how mucus congestion is created by casein: the 'rogue' casein amino acids that are digested trigger histamines in the body to fight the amino acids, and the body does this by creating mucus as a defence mechanism.

Among dairy products, milk is the worst because it causes more mucus in humans than any food you can eat. The casein in milk causes a thick dense mucus that clogs and irritates the body's entire respiratory system. This dense, gluey mucus coats the inside of the body and puts an enormous burden on the eliminative faculties of the delicate mucus membranes. This in turn invites disease and prevents the immune system from keeping harmful viruses and bacteria at bay.

Observe anybody who consumes half a pint of milk or more every day. You will notice that such people cough and sneeze and have more mucus congestion than people who do not consume milk.

Casein, which can only be obtained from dairy milk, is used in the manufacture of adhesives, binders, protective coatings, plastics (such as for knife handles and knitting needles), fabrics, and many other products.

> **Dairy milk contains many protein-allergens that cause allergic reactions. The two main allergens are whey and casein, and an individual may be allergic to either or both. The casein is the curd that forms when milk is left to sour, and the whey is the watery residue which is left after the curd is removed.**

Eat casein and your body produces histamines, then mucous. This sludge congests your organs. Give up all milk and dairy products for just one week and an internal "fog" will lift from your body.[24]

This is what happens: the casein mucus congestion lines the epithelial cells in our airways and allows invading viruses to pass our defences, causing infections such as colds and flu; plus many illnesses associated with the airways such as bronchitis, chest infections, coughs, aggravated asthma, and so on. Infections penetrate our defences because the tiny hairs that line the mucus membranes in our airways are clogged up. Fig. 1 shows how each epithelial cell contributes a few hairs:

Fig. 1
Epithelial cells lining the airways

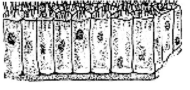

So when the hairs are clogged up with casein mucus they cannot catch and eject invading viruses, bacteria, dust and other debris. Healthy epithelial cells are able to undulate in a wave-like motion that carries debris out of the body. When the hairs are clogged with mucus, the undulating motion is ineffective.

The mucus membranes of people who consume dairy milk on a daily basis are in a perpetual state of mucosal congestion. Few people associate the ill effects caused by dairy milk because the milk tends to be consumed on a regular basis, providing a continuing state of mucosal congestion that is regarded as 'normal'.

- *Eighty percent of milk protein is casein, a tenacious glue and allergenic protein. Eat casein and you produce histamines, then mucous. The reaction is often delayed, occurring 12-15 hours after consumption…. By eliminating all dairy milk for one week, most people note the difference which includes better sleep, more energy, better bowel movements, clarity of thought, muscle, bone, and back pain relief…and goodbye to nasal congestion.*[6]

- *[Bovine] casein is very much less digestible than human casein. No addition we know of can render casein more digestible.*[93]

- *Casein is the major protein found in cow's milk (80-82%). Casein contains a high quantity of alpha Casein-a protein found only in animal milk, which is not easily digestible by humans. In fact, science shows that Casein in high amounts may actually delay gastric emptying.*[94]

- *Homogenization of milk reduces fat globule size and increases the facial area of the fat surface by a factor of 5-6. Simultaneously, the fat globules become coated with [bound with] a protein layer consisting of casein micelles and whey proteins.*[107]

- *The milk protein casein is similar in shape to the insulin-producing cells in the pancreas. Because the body may perceive casein as a foreign invader and attack It, It may also start to attack the pancreas cells having confused them for casein, again leading to diabetes.*[144]

The author Robert Cohen made the following comment in reference to 'Horizon's Organic Dairy' (a leading organic dairy producer in the USA):

'The healthiest [organic] milk from the healthiest [organic] cow is naturally loaded with lactoferrins, immunoglobulins, and growth hormones. Horizon's milk contains animal fat and cholesterol, dioxins, and bacteria. The amount of somatic cells (pus) in organic milk is lower than milk from nonorganic cows, but it's still dead white blood cells and dead bacteria. Ask yourself this question. Does organic human breast milk sound like a delicious drink for an adult human? Instinctively, most people know that there are substances in breast milk that are not intended for their adult bodies. The same goes for pig's milk, dog's milk, and cow's milk.

Some people may not be able to tolerate lactose, a milk sugar. One hundred percent of humans are allergic to casein, a milk protein. Eighty percent of the protein in Horizon's organic dairy products is casein, the same glue used to adhere a label to a bottle of beer. Eat casein and your body produces histamines, then mucous. This sludge congests your organs. Give up all milk and dairy products for just one week and an internal "fog" will lift from your body. Is genetically engineered milk dangerous? You bet!'[24]

Over fifty percent of casein (in milk generally) is not digested, depending on the physiology of the milk consumer, and is excreted. As explained in the chapter *The Lethal UHT Effect*, more casein is digested and absorbed with UHT milk, causing more congestion, illness, and disease compared to non-UHT milk.

According to the internet Wikipedia, a third of the casein in milk is bound with the tiny micronized fat globules that result from pasteurization and homogenization: *'The casein binds with the fat globules by coating the globules in casein'*.

The following table clarifies the position further: (see next page)

Is fat globule membrane partially denuded and then re-sealed (coated) by casein? *		
	Pasteurized milk	UHT milk
Homogenization ▶	Yes *	Yes * **(but more so)**
Heat treatment ▶	No *	Yes *

The above table shows that UHT homogenization breaks up and re-seals fat globules to a greater extent than pasteurized milk. It also shows that the pasteurization temperature used for regular milk is not hot enough to significantly affect casein. But the ultra-high temperatures of UHT cause casein to bind with other substances in milk.

'Heat treatment of HTST [regular pasteurized milk] *causes very little change in the fat globule membrane. However, excessively high pasteurization temperatures* [such as in UHT] *will partially denude the fat globule membranes.'*[123]

The critical point here is that far more fat globules are broken apart in UHT (compared to pasteurized milk) and as a result far more fat globules become partly covered in casein molecules. The consequence is that a greater number of casein-coated fat globules are digested, and hence a larger amount of harmful casein amino acids and peptides (two or more amino acids bounds together) are absorbed into the body.

The casein micelles (clumps of molecules) do not entirely coat the fat globule. Like chicken pox or craters on the moon, the globules are randomly covered in casein.

'The results strongly suggest that the proteins [mostly casein plus some whey] *of milk fat globule membrane are asymmetrically arranged in the membrane and that most of the protein-bound sialic acid is present on the external surface of milk fat globules.'*

As mentioned, the casein-coating effect helps keep the globules intact, and in so doing the casein 'seals' the globules, including any toxins and harmful substances that are bound with them. We have to realize that casein micelles (clumps of casein molecules) are very small, very plentiful, and very sticky. So when the fat globule membranes become ruptured, the rupture gets covered in casein micelles, thus sealing the rupture. The following diagram helps to illustrate this (see next page):

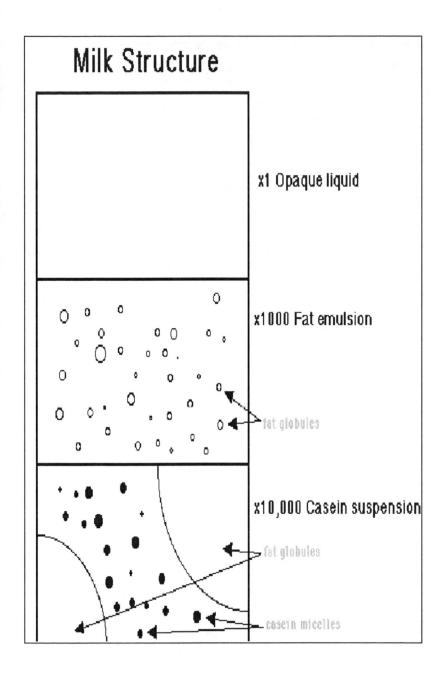

Milk Structure

x1 Opaque liquid

x1000 Fat emulsion

fat globules

x10,000 Casein suspension

fat globules

casein micelles

Casein micelles are clumps of casein molecules plus other substances.

It is known that UHT and regular pasteurized milk have similar amounts of casein. It is also known that casein is not denatured (broken down) merely by the heat treatment of UHT. But UHT sends more casein amino acids into the bloodstream for two reasons:

1. UHT homogenization makes a larger quantity of smaller fat globules with ruptured membranes. This in turn allows a larger number of fat globules to become coated by casein.

2. Casein is broken apart ('shredded') by the very high pressure of UHT homogenization, releasing clumps of casein molecules (micelles) that can bind with (coat) fat globules.

It is the combination of these two factors that serve to make UHT milk (including organic UHT) send larger amounts of harmful casein amino acids into the body to cause illness.

It should be remembered that casein itself causes harm to the body, and additionally it causes harm by sealing and enabling fat globules to carry harmful substances into the small intestine, thus increasing the amount of harmful substances that are absorbed into the body.

It is important to avoid giving dairy milk to children (particularly organic or nonorganic UHT milk) for the following reason:

In comparison to human milk, dairy milk contains 300% more casein and more than double the amount of total protein. Casein and lactoglobulin are the two main proteins in milk and they are unique in that they contain a perfect blend of amino acids, which is precisely what is needed during early infant growth. Human infants, however, double their mass on average 180 days after birth, whereas cows achieve the same feat in only 47 days. Dairy milk is therefore geared to meet the rapid growth requirements of cows, but is not suitable for humans. Casein also naturally stimulates thyroid function in infants and children, and as the thyroid is involved in many developmental processes, including the development of the nervous system, casein from other mammalian species could have adverse effects on the metabolic processes of infants.

To conclude this appendix, here is an edited extract from the book *Diet and Health* by Professor Walter J. Veith:

'The concentration of the enzyme rennin, that breaks down the casein, declines with age in all mammals, and by the time milk teeth develop it is virtually nonexistent in the human digestive tract. Without renin, the digestion of casein has to be carried out by the normal proteolytic enzymes which are not as efficient in breaking down casein. The presence of casein in the diet of mammals has also been linked to elevated cholesterol levels and various degenerative diseases such as arteriosclerosis (rabbits fed casein developed arteriosclerosis). Casein also produced higher cholesterol levels in humans, and seems to have an adverse effect on insulin secretion, thyrozine levels, gastrointestinal hormones and an adverse effect on calcium metabolism.'

***

Appendix B: IGF-1 – The Evidence

IGF-1 in milk may survive digestion:

- Anderle, P. et al, In Vitro Assessment of Intestinal IGF-1 Stability, Journal of Pharmaceutical Sciences, Jan. 2002, 91:1.

- Cooperative Research Centre, Women's and Children's Hospital, N. Adelaide, Australia, Journal of Endocrinology, 1995, 146:215-225.

- Kimura T. et al, Gastrointestinal absorption of recombinant human insulin-like growth factor-1 in rats, Journal of Pharmacology and Experimental Therapeutics, 1997, 283:611-618.

- Playford R. et al, Effect of luminal growth factor preservation on intestinal growth, Lancet, April 1993, 3(341):843-848.

- rBST Internal Review Team, rBST "Gaps Analysis" Report, Health Protection Branch, Health Canada, April 21, 1998.

- Xian C. et al, Degradation of IGF-1 in the adult rat gastrointestinal tract is limited by a specific antiserum or the dietary protein casein, Journal of Endocrinology, 1995, 146:215-225.

IGF-1 levels in milk may be at a high enough level to affect human health:

- Heaney R. et al, Dietary changes favorably affect bone remodelling in older adults, Journal of the American Dietetic Association, October 1999, 99:1229-1233.

- Holmes M. et al, Dietary correlates of plasma insulin-like growth factor 1 and insulin-like growth factor binding protein 3 concentrations, Cancer Epidemiology, Biomarkers and Prevention,, Sept. 2002, 11(9):852-861.

- Lahm H. et al, Growth regulation and co-stimulation of human colorectal cancer cell lines by insulin-like growth factor I, II and transforming growth factor alpha, British Journal of Cancer, March 1992, 65(3):341-346.

- Ma J. et al, Milk intake, circulating levels of IGF-1 and risk of colorectal cancer in men, Journal of the National Cancer Institute, Sept. 5, 2001, 93(17):1330-1336.

- Smith, G. et al, Editorial: Cancer and Insulin-like Growth Factor-1, British Medical Journal, Oct. 7, 2000, 321:847-848.

IGF-1 is associated with increased cancer risk:

- Chan J. et al, Plasma insulin-like growth factor-1 and prostate cancer risk: a prospective study, Science, Jan. 23, 1998, 279(5350):563-566.

- Giovannucci E. et al, A prospective study of plasma IGF-1 and binding protein-3 and risk of colorectal neoplasia in women, Cancer Epidemiology, Biomarkers & Prevention, 2000, 9:345-349.

- Hankinson S. et al, Circulating concentrations of insulin-like growth factor 1 and risk of breast cancer, Lancet, May 9, 1998, 351(9113):1393-1396.

- Lukanova A. et al, Circulating levels of IGF-1 and risk of ovarian cancer, International Journal of Cancer, October 20, 2002, 101(6):549-554.

- Moschos S. and Mantzoros C., The Role of the IGF System in Cancer: From Basic to Clinical Studies and Clinical Applications, Oncology, Nov. 4, 2002, 63(4):317-332.

- Yu H. and Rohan T., Role of the Insulin-Like Growth Factor Family in Cancer Development and Progression, Journal of the National Cancer Institute, Sept. 20, 2000, 92(18):1472-1489.

- Yu H. et al, Plasma levels of IGF-1 and lung cancer risk: a case-control analysis, Journal of the National Cancer Institute, Jan. 20, 1999, 91(2):151-156.

For the leading causes of death in the USA please see next page ▶

Ten biggest causes of death in the USA (Heart disease is the biggest)	
1. Heart disease	Milk products contribute to clogged arteries
2. *Cancer*	***Milk provides IGF-1 (cancer-causing hormones), toxins, and harmful calcification, all of which increase the risk of cancer.***
3. Cerebrovascular diseases	Milk provides damaged proteins and heavy metals which affect the brain. Milk also increases the risk of strokes.
4. Chronic lower respiratory diseases	Milk provides casein which causes respiratory diseases.
5. Unintentional injuries	Avoid milk and you will feel better, be healthier, think more clearly, and be less likely to have accidents.
6. Diabetes mellitus	Milk is the biggest dietary cause of diabetes.
7. Influenza and pneumonia	Milk lowers immunity and provides casein which impairs whole respiratory system.
8. Alzheimer's disease	Milk provides damaged proteins and heavy metals which affect the brain.

9. Kidney inflammation/disease	Milk causes kidney disease arising from casein which impairs kidney function. Milk also causes harmful calcification in the kidneys.
10. Septicemia (disease caused by the spread of bacteria and toxins in the bloodstream)	Milk, more than any other kind of food, feeds toxins to the bloodstream, while simultaneously lowering immunity.

Source for first column: U.S. National Center for Health Statistics, 'Health', United States, 2005.

The following edited extract is taken from the website www.notmilk.com:

CANCER FUEL

Most cow's milk has measurable quantities of herbicides, pesticides, dioxins (up to 200 times the safe levels), up to 52 powerful antibiotics (perhaps 53, with LS-50), blood, pus, bacteria, viruses, fat, cholesterol, scores of allergens, and feces (cow's milk can have traces of anything the cow ate... including such things as radioactive fallout from nuke testing – the 50's strontium-90 problem).

Milk also has a total of 59 hormones, and one is a powerful GROWTH hormone called Insulin-like Growth Factor ONE (IGF-1). By a freak of nature it is identical in cows and humans. Consider this hormone to be a "fuel cell" for any cancer... (the medical world says IGF-1 is a key factor in the rapid growth and proliferation of breast, prostate and colon cancers, and we suspect that most likely it will be found to promote ALL cancers).

IGF-1 is a normal part of ALL milk... the newborn is SUPPOSED to grow quickly! What makes the 50% of obese American consumers think they need MORE growth? Consumers don't think anything about it because they do not have a clue to the problem... nor do most of our doctors.

*** *

Appendix C: Other Aspects of Milk

This appendix is included for the sake of completeness as they relate to dairy milk generally, whether or not organic or UHT.

Irritable Bowel Syndrome

It is estimated that about a quarter of all adults suffer periodically from IBS (Irritable Bowel Syndrome), causing a multitude of digestive disorders. Stress used to be thought of as a major cause of IBS, but it is now thought that dairy milk is the biggest cause.

The lactose, indigestible protein, and antibiotics in the milk all combine to provide a ready-made cocktail for IBS. *Some kinds of bacteria in dairy milk are able to survive pasteurization, causing Johne's Disease, Crohns Disease, and IBS...*[6] By simply giving up dairy milk, most people find that IBS disappears.

Ear infections

Ear infections are another major cause of disease from dairy milk:

- *Milk allergies ...are the leading cause of chronic ear infections that plague up to 40% of all children under the age of six.*[45]

- *Cows milk allergy is associated with recurrent otitis media (ear infection) during childhood.*[46]

- *Concerning ear infections, you just don't see this painful condition among infants and children who aren't getting cow's milk into their systems.*[47]

- *Cow's milk is the primary cause of recurrent ear infections in children. It has also been linked to insulin dependent diabetes, rheumatoid arthritis, infertility, and leukemia.*[40]

In the book *Killers Within* the authors reveal that *Staphylococcus Aureus* is the most common infection of dairy cows. Typical symptoms in humans include nausea, vomiting, diarrhoea, abdominal cramps, and fever. Bacterial toxins are easily passed from cows to humans in milk, and are not always destroyed by pasteurization. On page 30, the authors write: *Staphlococcus Aureus bacteria are so virulent that very few are needed to do the job...it's the most successful of all bacterial pathogens and the number one cause of hospital infections in the world.*[3]

Iron Deficiency

Iron is needed for good bone marrow formation and therefore has a direct effect on body growth. During the first 6 months of life, babies are usually protected against developing iron deficiency due to the stores of iron built up in their bodies before they are born. However, when over six months old, as infants continue to undergo significant growth, they usually do not take in enough iron through breast milk alone.

If consuming dairy milk, iron deficiency in a child or infant is exacerbated in three ways:

1. Dairy milk contains virtually no iron and therefore contributes nothing towards the prevention of anaemia. The trace amount of iron that dairy milk contains (less than one milligram per quart) is poorly absorbed. Some of the indigestible protein in milk binds with the iron which then leaves the

body without being absorbed into the bloodstream.

2. Dairy milk makes an infant less interested in eating other foods that are good for body growth and that provide better sources of iron. This is because dairy milk is filling and takes longer to digest, thus satiating feelings of hunger for more nutritious food.

3. Dairy milk causes some infants to lose iron from their intestines through intestinal bleeding (the harsh casein in milk irritates the delicate lining of the baby's intestines). This bleeding is insidious and usually not sufficiently severe to be noticed in stools, but enough to cause anaemia. It is estimated that half the iron-deficiency in infants in the USA is from cow-milk induced intestinal bleeding!

UHT milk (whether or not organic) is worse because, as explained in Appendix A, more casein enters the bloodstream, and this in turn makes intestinal bleeding worse than otherwise.

Many studies have been carried out that show how dairy milk causes intestinal bleeding. Here are extracts from some of these studies:

Milk consumption has been shown to cause intestinal bleeding, resulting in low hemoglobin count. The result: weakness, depression, irritability.[6]

Babies who are fed whole cow's milk during the second six months of life may experience a 30% increase in intestinal blood loss and a significant loss of iron in their stools.[53]

Children with iron deficiency had a higher intake of cow's milk compared to those with sufficient iron.

Intake of cow's milk is significantly higher in children with iron deficiency.[54]

Cow's milk-induced intestinal bleeding is a well-recognized cause of rectal bleeding in infancy. In all cases, bleeding resolved completely after instituting a cow's milk-free diet.[55]

Significant rectal bleeding is the most common symptom in cow's milk allergy.[56]

Cow's milk has been linked to a variety of health problems, including haemoglobin loss, mood swings, depression, and irritability.[57]

The association with anaemia and acute intestinal bleeding in infants is known to all physicians.[9]

Contamination

Dairy milk causes a multitude of diseases. Its derivative dairy products contain no fibre or complex carbohydrates and are mostly laden with saturated fat and rancid cholesterol. Dairy milk (including organic milk) is contaminated with cow's blood and pus cells, which are often not neutralized through pasteurization. Virtually all dairy cows are given drugs, hormones and antibiotics to make them produce plenty of milk for as long as possible. Also, the grass (if any) and food they eat is frequently contaminated with filth and farm waste, giving rise to E. coli, salmonella, and listeria, leading to food poisoning and illness in humans who consume dairy milk.

In a major study in the USA over 76% of pasteurized milk transported by bulk tankers was found to be contaminated with E. coli bacteria.

In addition to farm waste, dairy cows are increasingly being fed disease-ridden commercial and domestic waste as a way of cutting down on land-fill costs. *'Feeding waste products* [to cows] *has some positive economic impacts for the milk producer. If they can buy waste products for less than they can buy traditional feed ingredients, it will reduce their cost of milk production. The alternative of feeding much of the material to livestock would be to landfill it, and that has some significant costs to society.'* [41]

Feedgrains destined for livestock (including dairy cows) are usually sprayed heavily with herbicides and pesticides. These are hydrocarbons, the repeated ingestion of which may raise the risk of birth defects or cancer.

These pesticides, herbicides, hormones, drugs and antibiotics are passed into the milk and *are not eliminated with pasteurization.* Furthermore, all lactating mammals eliminate some of their toxic waste through their milk!

Disease

Dairy milk and dairy products are linked to a long list of illnesses. In particular, antigenic proteins in cow's milk can 'leak' into the bloodstream of a milk consumer through the intestinal lining and incite allergic reactions in lungs and joints – exacerbating asthma and rheumatoid arthritis, among other things.

Here are a few comments from physicians and scientists regarding diseases caused by dairy milk:

- *Certain foods trigger the symptoms of* **rheumatoid arthritis***, and eliminating these foods sometimes causes even long-standing symptoms to improve or even remit entirely. It's important to avoid the problem foods completely, as even a small amount can cause symptoms. All dairy products should be avoided: skim or* *whole milk, goat's milk, cheese, yogurt, cream, etc.*[42]

- *Milk's biological purpose is to promote rapid growth in infant cows. It makes biological sense that its nutrients and hormonal effects might also promote the growth of cancer cells.*[43]

- *There is a colossal amount of information linking the consumption of milk to arthritis...and a multitude of other problems as documented by Hannah Allen, Alec Burton, Viktoras Kulvinsdas, F.M. Pottenger, Herbert M, Shelton, and N.L. Walker, among others.*[44]

- *From 1988 to 1993 there were over 2,700 articles dealing with [dairy] milk recorded in the "Medicine" archives... There is no lack of scientific information on the subject. I reviewed over 500 articles. They were only slightly less than horrifying...none of the authors spoke of cow's milk as an excellent food. The main focus seemed to be on intestinal colic, intestinal irritation, bleeding, anemia, allergic reactions, viral infection with bovine leukemia, childhood diabetes, and contamination of milk by blood and pus cells, as well as a variety of chemicals and insecticides, were also discussed.*[9]

The list of ailments cited by medical writers in relation to dairy milk is almost too long to publish. Here are just a few in no particular order: constipation, obesity, heart disease, several types of cancer (including ovarian, lung, and breast cancer), colitis, tonsillitis arthritis, sinusitis, asthma, infant anemia, leukemia, diabetes, gastrointestinal bleeding, atherosclerosis, salmonella, diarrhoea, abdominal cramps, migraine, colds, and many other diseases.

Prostate cancer, for example, is strongly associated with dairy milk as evidenced by many studies. Peer-reviewed research published in mainstream medical journals shows beyond any doubt that dairy milk is by far the biggest dietary cause of prostate cancer.[7]

Similarly, there is a strong link between milk consumption and breast cancer. Calcium from milk causes harmful calcification in the breasts leading to breast cancer.[7]

And let's not forget BSE (known as 'mad cow disease'). The fact that humans can catch BSE from eating cooked cow's meat has been proven. When it comes to BSE and dairy milk, the jury is still out!

Every year several cases of mad cow disease are reported in North America. The USA Consumer's Union states:

Mad cow disease is a fatal, brain-wasting affliction, which can be passed on to humans by eating tainted beef. Consumers Union has serious concerns about the effectiveness of the U.S. mad cow surveillance program including its failure to use the most sensitive and up-to-date testing methods that are used in Europe and Japan. Just as troublesome is the fact that the [US] government does not have mandatory recall authority and refuses to publicize the names of the retailers that are selling the tainted meat. Source: www.consumersunion.org.

Crohn's Disease deserves a special mention. Scientists at Liverpool University, UK, announced in December 2007 that milk may be contributing to Crohn's Disease. The Liverpool University research shows that a bacteria called **Mycobacterium Paratuberculosis** (abbreviated to MAP) is widely present in pasteurized milk – yes, *pasteurized* milk.

By consuming milk, MAP acts to weaken the immune system by preventing white blood cells from killing e.coli. This in turn allows Crohn's Disease to develop in humans. *'It is thought that the* Mycobacteria *make their way into the body's system via cows' milk and other dairy products.'*[128]

Professor John Hermon-Taylor, the UK's leading expert on Crohn's Disease, has called for a mass vaccination of cattle against becoming infected with MAP so as to help prevent Crohn's Disease in milk consumers.

Research carried out in 2000 by the UK's Food Standards Agency found that 2.1 percent of *pasteurized* milk contained MAP.

In the USA, where the authorities are more lenient in the disease-control of cows, it is thought that 5 percent of pasteurized milk is infected with MAP. A similar picture emerges in other countries.

The USDA has found that Bovine Johne's Disease (the bovine equivalent of Crohn's Disease) has become an enormous problem for US cattle farmers. A USDA survey (Johne's Disease on U.S. Dairy Operations) found that 40% of large farms (with more than 200 animals) contain animals infected with Bovine Johne's Disease, and over 20% of small farms contain infected cows.

Currently, there is no published research that specifically compares the incidence of Bovine Johne's Disease in organic and nonorganic dairy farms. A comparison would be interesting given that the MAP bacteria is spread through cow-pats and animal farm waste. Organic cows are more likely to come into contact with such waste (because it is widely used as fertilizer), and they are more likely to acquire MAP infection by virtue of not receiving regular antibiotic medication. The incidence of MAP may therefore be higher in organic pasteurized milk compared to regular pasteurized milk.

'Some research suggests the widespread use of animal manure, when composted improperly, results in a higher occurrence of pathogens than conventional farming.'[1]

Appendix D: Unhealthy UHT homogenization

The purpose of UHT homogenization is to ensure that the cream in milk does not separate and that a uniform texture is maintained indefinitely. This is necessary because UHT milk is designed for non-refrigerated storage of up to 6 months at ambient temperature.

Just about all modern UHT plants homogenize the milk first, followed by pasteurization because this method is found to be more economical and efficient. Technically, this is known as the *UHT Indirect Method*.

(Note: The older, less efficient *UHT Direct Method* is, if anything, worse for health because the milk is first pasteurized and then sprayed into a hot steam chamber. This causes greater molecular damage to milk and has other detrimental affects).

The time interval between homogenization and pasteurization is a matter of seconds or minutes because it's all part of one continuous flow process.

Here is a brief description of how UHT milk is processed in a modern UHT milk plant:[117]

- First, the raw milk is heated to 75°C and then homogenized at very high pressure. Homogenization is a process by which fat globules in milk are made much smaller. Milk is forced under high pressure through tiny holes/tubes. The higher the pressure, the greater the breakdown of fat globules.

- The milk then continues along piped conduits to a second heating section where it is heated to 137°C or more, depending on the type of plant and method used. Heating is performed by hot water in a closed hot-water circuit. After heating (i.e. ultra-high-temperature pasteurizing) the milk cools down as it is piped towards packaging or intermediate storage before packaging.

The number of fat globules in regular *pasteurized* milk is about 10,000 greater than in untreated milk. The number of fat globules in *UHT* milk is nearly 20,000 greater than in untreated milk.

This results in a decrease in the average diameter of the fat globules, an increase in their number and an increase of their total surface area. (Many smaller globules have a bigger *total* surface area than fewer bigger globules).

Other milk solids like casein and whey protein are also broken up during homogenization.

So there is a big increase in the density and compactness of fat globules, and a big reduction in the mean diameter of the globules.

Technically milk is a colloidal suspension of water that contains a variety of particles (milk solids). The main solids are protein, lactose and fat, each taking up about a third of the milk-solid volume (very roughly).

Before milk is pasteurized and homogenized, each kind of milk solid is mostly suspended separately in the milk (they are not physically or chemically bound together at this stage).

But UHT homogenization, followed by the very high temperatures of UHT pasteurization, serve to break down and bring together many of these solids. Here is what happens:

1. UHT homogenization breaks down the protein and fat. Whey proteins are damaged and casein

protein is broken apart. Fat globules are ripped apart (the outer membranes of the globules are torn open as a result of bigger globules being smashed into smaller globules).

2. Soon after homogenization, the milk is ultra heated to a very high temperature (nearly 50% higher than boiling point). The high pressure of pasteurization prevents the milk from bubbling up as it would on a domestic cooker. The ultra high heat breaks the homogenized fat down to even smaller fat globules. When any kind of fat is heated (as in cooking for example) the fat globules are broken down to smaller fat globules.

3. The high heat treatment binds some of the milk solids with some of the fat globules. It also binds fat molecules with any toxins that may be present in milk. Remember that at this point the membranes of the fat globules have been ruptured by homogenization, so it is easier for the globules to bind with anything in its proximity. Heat has the effect of mixing and binding everything together (think how ingredients become completely mixed when cooked in a saucepan).

4. In this unfolding drama 'casein enters centre stage'. Casein is sticky and there is lots of it in milk. Some fragments and molecules of milk solids bind with casein (e.g. damaged whey proteins and lactose); others bind with the ruptured fat globules.

5. As the milk cools the casein and fat 'coalesce', making the casein coat the fat globules (see Appendix A for a detailed explanation). So casein acts to seal the ruptured membranes of fat globules, and in so doing seals in any substances that are bound with the globules such as IGF-1,

toxins, and sex hormones. So, for example, damaged whey proteins are bound with casein, and then the casein in turn is bound with fat globules.

6. When the milk is consumed many of the tiny micronized fat globules are easily digested by virtue of their small size and by virtue of being evenly spread in the milk as an emulsion (this is how the digestive system likes to receive food). As a result, more of the fat globule's cargo than otherwise (toxins, casein, damaged whey proteins, and IGF-1 hormones) manage to penetrate the intestinal wall and enter the body.

7. These harmful substances can enter the bloodstream and can then be distributed to many parts of the body to cause illness and disease. This is how casein is carried to organs, tissues, and the respiratory system to cause congestion and illness. This is how damaged whey proteins enter the brain to cause brain disease (see chapter 'Brain Disease'). This is how galactose (a component of lactose) is distributed to places like the eyes to cause cataracts. And this is how heavy metals and dioxins can be taken to places in the body where they can cause cancer and brain disease.

Here are some extracts from some of the research explaining how casein and whey proteins stick to the newly formed fat globules after homogenization:

- *A greater number of smaller particles possess more total* <u>*surface area*</u> *than a smaller number of larger ones, and the original fat globule membranes cannot completely cover them. Casein micelles* [strands of molecules] *are attracted to the newly-exposed fat surfaces;*

nearly one-third of the micelles in the milk end up participating in this new membrane structure. The casein weighs down the globules and interferes with the clustering that accelerated separation. The exposed fat globules are briefly vulnerable to certain enzymes present in milk, which could break down the fats and produce rancid flavors. To prevent this, the enzymes are inactivated by pasteurizing the milk immediately before or after homogenization.(Source: Wikipedia).

- *The fat globules that are formed during homogenization are covered with plasma proteins to coat the increased surface area caused by homogenization.*[109]

- *During homogenization, the fat globule membrane is disrupted, leaving the globule with only some of its original membrane. Casein micelles* [clumps of molecules] *adsorb on* [stick to] *the uncovered surface and assist in globule stabilization and water binding. A heat treatment* [i.e. pasteurization] *of the milk prior to adsorption results in a complete membrane, possibly even thicker. Before heat treatment, the fat globule's membrane prevents extensive protein interactions, but once heat is applied, the casein micelle and whey protein structures change and adsorb on the fat.*[110]

Remember that following homogenization, the fat globules become more compact and densely packed throughout the milk. They are therefore in closer proximity to other milk solids, and to any toxins that may be present.

Compared to regular pasteurized milk, more damaged milk solids, toxins, and harmful substances bind with the micronized fat globules in UHT for three reasons:

1. The non-refrigerated storage of UHT milk, which can be for several weeks or months, *increases the amount of damaged milk solids (and toxins) that bind with fat globules*. However, this largely depends on storage conditions (length of time and storage temperatures). See *Appendix E: Effects of UHT Storage* for more information.

2. With UHT, there is a *greater breakdown of milk solids*. This in turn results in more milk-solid fragments binding with the newly micronized fat globules.

3. With UHT, fat globules are deliberately made smaller as a way of avoiding cream separation at anytime in the future. This allows UHT milk to be stored for up to 6 months at ambient temperature with no separation of cream and with no change in uniformity of milk texture.

The homogenization of milk is a well studied science in the dairy industry. It is known that the greater the micronization of fat globules, the more they will bind with damaged milk solids, toxins, and harmful substances.

It is a fact of chemistry that when you heat any kind of fat, the fat globules are broken up and made smaller. Later, as the fat cools down, the fat globules will tend to coalesce back into bigger globules.

But with UHT the fat globules do not coalesce back into bigger globules for two reasons: (i) molecular changes caused by homogenization & ultra-high heat treatment prevent coalescence, and (ii) the fat globules become coated with casein, thus preventing coalescence into bigger globules.

Appendix E: Effects of UHT Storage

UHT milk is typically stored without refrigeration for several weeks (or even months) before consumption. This has a dramatic effect on the nutritional value, composition, and quality of the milk. This constitutes a major difference between UHT milk (*including organic UHT*) and regular pasteurized milk.

Disconcertingly, when you buy UHT milk and see the 'sell-by-date' printed on the carton or container, you still have no way of knowing how old the milk is. Some milk companies may put 3 month sell-by-dates on the cartons, others 6 months, and still others 9 months for sterilized milk, so you have no way of calculating the true age of such milk.

The detrimental effects of storage depend on the length of time stored and the storage temperature. Typically, the storage temperatures are likely to be those of a warehouse or supermarket shelf. Generally, the longer the period of UHT storage the more significant the increase in acidity, galactose, and degradation of the milk.

An increase in milk acidity due to UHT storage is harmful because this increases acidity levels in the blood. This in turn triggers harmful hormonal levels in the blood which try to neutralize the increased acidity level.

An increase in milk galactose levels due to UHT storage is harmful because high galactose levels cause illness (see 'Galactose' chapter). Milk is already super rich in galactose and UHT storage can exacerbate this.

An increase in milk degradation due to UHT storage is harmful because it increases the level of denatured whey proteins (see 'Brain Disease' chapter) and it greatly reduces the nutritional value of the milk.

Here is a small selection of the many research papers showing the harmful effects of UHT storage:

Increase in harmful acidity

- In all samples [of the milk being tested] acidity increased from day one. The increase in acidity of the samples of UHT treated milk and whole milk powder during storage period of 90 days might be due to the formation of lactic acid by lactic acid bacteria.[73][2]

- One of the most important factors involved in increasing the acidity of milk samples during storage is the storage condition; milk treated at ultra high temperature can be stored for a certain period of time. During storage milk undergoes various changes; therefore, storage conditions may have a pronounced effect on titratable [total] acidity of the stored milk. For example, storage temperature determines the microbial activity leading to the formation of lactic acids. Rerkrai et al. [1986] found that titratable acidity varies due to prevailing storage conditions. Storage time and temperature have a great effect on the acidity of the stored milk as reported by Kocak and Zadow [1985].[76]

- Titratable [total] acidity increased gradually from 0.135 to 0.177 and 0.192 after 33 days [Adhikari and Singhal 1992]. Ito [1985] confirmed the increase in acidity of UHT milk during storage. Gorner et al. [1977] observed a gradual increase in titratable acidity at an irregular rate and attributed this behaviour to the changes in milk protein.[77]

- The acidity of UHT increased from day 30 to day 60 during the entire storage period... The pH values decreased [acidity increased] again from 60 days storage to 90 days.[102] Author's comment: no pH figures can be given for stored UHT milk because the pH figures will depend on storage temperatures, and storage period. Therefore, acidity levels will vary greatly from carton to carton and from retail outlet to retail outlet.

Increase in harmful galactose

- The changes in the concentration of...sugar phosphates in UHT milk were studied for 120 days. An increase in galactose... was found, which was larger as the temperature of storage increased.[121]

- An increase in galactose was found which was larger as the [UHT] temperature of storage increased. Changes in galactose during storage at 30°C...may have potential detrimental consequences to milk stability.[83] Note that temperatures of 30°C are often reached during transportation; also non-refrigerated supermarket shelves can easily reach 30°C.

- Storage effects on levels of galactose in UHT milk stored at 10°C to 30°C for 120 days were investigated. An increase in galactose was observed, the increase being more pronounced at higher storage temperatures. Milk batches with high proteolytic [breakdown of protein] activity showed a considerable increase in galactose.[84]

Increase in milk degradation

- Scientists in Australia, a country with a huge dairy industry, have taken the lead in researching UHT milk. A 2002 paper discusses how UHT processing and subsequent storage causes several changes affecting the shelf life of UHT milk. The changes include: whey protein denaturation, protein-protein interaction, lactose-protein interaction, isomerisation of lactose, and formation of insoluble substances. According to the authors Datta and Deeth, these changes *"ultimately reduce the quality and limit the shelf life of UHT through development of off flavors, fat separation, age gelation and sedimentation. Nevertheless the milk remains "commercially stable."* [118]

- *Degradation of caseins and whey proteins…were studied in six batches of commercial UHT milk during storage at room temperature. Extensive proteolytic degradation of the micellar fractions and severe changes in the electrophoretic pattern of the proteins present in the serum fractions were observed in all the batches.* [119]

- Some research is showing that storage times of UHT milk exacerbate the content of saturated fat: *'UHT milk samples processed at 140°C for 2 sec were stored at 9°, 15°, 25°, 35°, 45° and 55°C and analysed for free fatty acids (FFA) released as a result of lipid hydrolysis. The levels of FFA in the UHT milk increased….after 16 weeks of storage. At 55°C, FFA level increased to 5.68 µeq/ml after only 12 weeks of storage. The GLC analysis of FFA showed that the major contributors to the increase in saturated fatty acids were C_4-C_{12} fatty acids which increased* *from the initial value of 2.66 (mole %) to…. 5.02 (mole %) after 16 weeks of storage at 25°, 35° and 45°C, respectively. At 55°C, the increase was 5.55 (mole %) after 12 weeks of storage.*[120]

- Several studies of stored UHT milk[118] show that milk contains endocrine disrupting substances that leak from the plastic of the containers, or the plastic lining the containers. Even when kept cold, plastic will leach some chemicals into the liquid it contains; filling plastic-lined containers with superheated milk or subjecting liquid-filled containers to high heat is a recipe for the release of phthalates and similar substances. Levels of these compounds in the samples studied did not achieve *'the maximum leached level allowed by law. The impact these compounds may have on organisms and human beings needs to be further studied, especially with regard to accumulation, degradation and possible effects within the endocrine system.'*[118]

- *'The nutritive value of UHT milk can be reduced during storage after packaging…Water soluble vitamins and proteins are adversely affected.'*[116]

- *'Some of the vitamins, e.g. folic acid and vitamin C, are oxidationsensitive, and their losses occur mainly during storage* [of UHT milk] *due to a high oxygen content in the milk or in the package. However, milk is not a good source of vitamin C and folic acid, as the content is far below the recommended daily intake.'*[117]

Appendix F: The Nutritional Aspects Of Organic Milk – A Review Of The Evidence

This appendix reflects the information put out by organic milk lobbyists generally, and serves to give the reader both sides of the 'argument'.

The organic milk lobbyist says:

Several scientific studies have demonstrated the nutritional benefits of organic milk. They show that organic milk generally contains higher levels of beneficial nutrients and vitamins than milk from non-organic cows. The studies have found that organic milk contains higher levels of beneficial compounds in the milk fats, particularly short-chain omega-3 essential fatty acids, as well as vitamin E and the antioxidant beta-carotene (which the body converts to vitamin A). Higher levels of the antioxidants lutein and zeaxanthine have also been found in milk from cows that eat a grass-based diet typical of organic farming.

Author's comment:

Please see the chapters in this book titled "Nutrition" and "The More Nutritious Myth" for the evidence showing that organic milk is not more nutritious than nonorganic milk.

The organic milk lobbyist says:

The nutritional benefits of organic milk can be explained by the diets of organic cows. Organic cows eat a much more natural diet mostly consisting of fresh grass and clover (forage). In comparison, non-organic dairy farmers are allowed to use more grain-based (concentrate) feed containing cereals, malze and protein supplements. These diets increase milk yields but also affect the nutritional composition of the milk.

Author's comment:

Clearly, a cohort of carefully controlled cows fed a rich diet of fresh grass and clover throughout the year are going to produce more nutritious milk, whether or not the cows are organic. But the vast majority of organic cows do not live in showcase experimental farms. Hence virtually all organic milk is no different to nonorganic milk when it comes to nutritional content. There is no evidence to show that random samples of organic milk taken from random supermarket shelves are any more nutritious than nonorganic milk.

The organic milk lobbyist says:

The Vitamins and antioxidants in organic milk have a range of nutritional benefits, including cancer and disease prevention.

Author's comment:

This argument can be put forward by just about any kind of food producer. In reality, just about any kind of food can be said to have vitamins and antioxidants that 'have a range of nutritional benefits, including cancer and disease prevention.' Of course, what counts is the quality and amount of nutrients, and how well they are digested. As explained in this book, there is no evidence showing that organic milk (as purchased randomly from a retailer) gives a milk consumer a higher amount of vitamins and antioxidants compared to nonorganic milk.

The organic milk lobbyist says:

Some studies have shown that organic milk contains higher levels of short-chain omega-3 fatty acids

(ALA). Research has also identified a higher content of the omega-6 fatty acids, conjugated linoleic acid (CLA) and linoleic acid, as well as a more beneficial (lower) ratio of omega-3 and omega-6 in organic milk compared to nonorganic milk.

Author's comment:

Please see the chapter in this book titled "*The More Nutritious Myth*" for the evidence showing that organic milk is not more nutritious than nonorganic milk in terms of fatty acids. Organic milk lobbyists do quote studies showing that it is more nutritious. However, it should be remembered that none of the studies quoted are based on random samples of organic milk taken from a random selection of retailers. The studies were either based on carefully controlled cohorts of cows or they were based on testing raw milk before it was pasteurized. Any small differences in the nutritional content of organic and nonorganic milk are largely rendered irrelevant by the process of pasteurization and homogenization which greatly degrades nutritional value. It should also be remembered that there are just as many studies (if not more) showing that organic milk is not more nutritious.

For example, in April 2008 sixty-six dairy and veterinary scientists from just about every major university in the USA signed an open letter saying that consumers were being misled by emotional advertising and that "*there was no nutritional difference between conventional and organic milk*". The letter cited a 2007/8 study of more than 200 organic and nonorganic milk samples taken from retail stores across the USA. "*Tests showed the same nutrient content for both types of milk.*" [162]

Further Reading

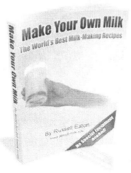

Make Your Own Milk
The world's best milk-making recipes
For more information please go to:
www.about-milk.info

This unique ebook has brought together the world's best recipes for making non-dairy milk at home. Now you can enjoy super-delicious and nutritious milk whenever you like. These milk recipes cannot be found anywhere else. In a matter of minutes you can make milk quickly and easily, without using any special milk-making apparatus. Once you start making your own milk you will never want to go back to buying commercial milk. *Make Your Own Milk* makes it easy to switch from dairy to non-dairy milk, saving you time and money and improving your health.

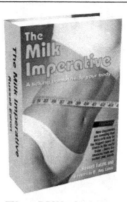

The Milk Imperative
A ticking bomb inside your body
For more information please go to:
www.about-milk.info

New discoveries are revealing that dairy milk may be the biggest cause of illness in the world today. *The Milk Imperative* breaks new ground by revealing exactly how dairy milk causes osteoporosis and prostate cancer, backed up with the latest scientific studies. This book is sending shock waves through the dairy industry, and whether or not you consume dairy milk *The Milk Imperative* will change your life forever.

About the Author

Russell Eaton was born in London and mostly grew up in Ecuador. He then moved back to England where he worked in the computer industry for many years. He has a *Higher National Diploma in Business Studies*, University of Wales, and is now an established author with 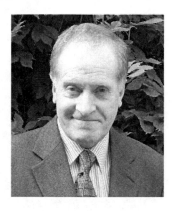 books relating to travel, health, and property. With a life-long interest in health and nutrition he says: *'Organic Milk Myth' was a book waiting to be written because the supporting evidence is now so overwhelming. All types of dairy milk are bad for health, but by far the worst are the two kinds of milk covered in the book, that is, organic and UHT pasteurized milk.*

Details of other books by Russell Eaton can be obtained by going to www.deliveredonline.com.

References

1. Bishop, Rusty, Ph.D., Director, Center for Dairy Research, Department of Food Science, University of Wisconsin – Madison, USA, *Science Behind Reported Benefits of Organic Milk,* Oct. 2007.

2. Stewart, K L. 2007, *Is the organic milk glass half full or half empty?* NutraUSAIngredients.com, January 30.

3. Mark J. Plotkin & Michael Shnayerson, *The Killers Within: The Deadly Rise of Drug Resistant Bacteria*, Back Bay Books, Sep. 2003, ISBN 0316735663.

4. Professor Ken Green and Dr Chris Foster, Manchester Business School, UK, published by DEFRA, Department of Environment, Farming and Rural Affairs, 2007.

5. Journal of the National Institute of Health, 1991,3.

6. Robert Cohen, *Milk A-Z*, 2001, Argus Publishing, ISBN 0965919684; and Science, vol. 249, august 24, 1990.

7. Russell Eaton, *The Milk Imperative*, 2006, www.milkimperative.com.

8. Journal of the National Institute of Health, 1991-3.

9. Robert Cohen, Milk – *The Deadly Poison*, Argus Publishing, January 1, 1998, ISBN: 0965919609.

10. Molecular Cell Endocrinology, March, 99(2).

11. Journal of Cellular Physiology, January, 1994, 158(1).

12. European Journal of Cancer, 29A (16), 1993.

13. Experimental Cell Research, March, 1994, 211(1).

14. Science, Vol. 259, January 29, 1993.

15. Science, vol. 279, January 23, 1998.

16. The Lancet, vol. 351, May 9, 1998.

17. Journal of the National Cancer Institute, vol. 91, no. 2, January 20, 1999.

18. International Journal of Cancer, 2000 Aug. 87:4.

19. Rosemary Hoskins, Food Fact no. 2, A Safe Alliance Publication, 1998.

20. Dr. Sarfaraz K. Niazi, PhD pharmaceutical sciences, University of Illinois, USA.

21. Yu, H, Rohan, Role of the insulin-like growth factor family in cancer development and progression, Journal of the National Cancer Institute, Sept. 20, 2000, 92(18):1472-1481).

22. (Kimura, T, Murakawa Y, Ohno M, Higaki K, Gastrointestinal absorption of recombinant human insulin-like growth factor-1 in rats, Journal of Pharmacology and Experimental Therapeutics, July 1997, 283:611-618).

23. Patricia Alonso-Toledo, Studies of …Organic Production Systems, Dept of Food Science, Uppsala, 2003.

24. Robert Cohen, Executive Director, Dairy Education Board, 201-871-5871, www.notmilk.com.

25. Prof. Rusty Bishop, Ph.D., Director, Center for Dairy Research, Dept. of Food Science, University of Wisconsin – Madison, USA, Science Behind Reported Benefits of Organic Milk, October 12, 2007.

26. Ganmaa D, et al, Incidence and mortality of testicular and prostatic cancers in relation to world dietary practices. *Int.J.Cancer*, 2002;98:262-7.

27. Dr. Leo Galland's Drug-Nutrient Interactions Workshop Software from Allergy Research Group 800-545-9960.

28. Janowski T., Mammary secretion of oestrogens in the cow, Domest Anim Endocrinol. 2002 Jul; 23(1-2): 125-37.

29. Sharon Gerdes, technical consultant for Dairy Management, which represents U.S. dairy farmers.

30. Karen Collins, RD, *Nutrition Notes, August 2006, American Institute for Cancer Research, Washington, D.C.*

31. The 'Food Standards Agency' and the 'Joint Health Claims Initiative'. These bodies are responsible for investigating and approving health claims, reported in The Sunday Times, UK, p. 10 News, Nov. 6, 2005).

32. Ghidini, S, et al. 2005. Comparison of contaminant and residue levels in organic and conventional milk and meat products from Northern Italy. Food Additives and Contaminants 22(1):9-14.

33. Vallone, L, et al. 2006. Aflatoxins in organic milk and dairy products. Veterinary Research Communications 30(Suppl 1):369-370.

34. *Acta Paediatrica*, 1999 Dec, 88:12.

35. Nicholas, Samsidis, MS *Homogenized - How Homogenized Milk Triggers Heart and Circulatory Disease*, Park City Pr; June 1994.

36. Survey of Mortality Rates and Food Consumption Statistics of 24 Countries, Medical Hypothesis, 7:907-918, 1981.

37. European Journal of Clinical Nutrition, 48, 1994.

38. Circulation, 1993; 88,6.

39. Alternative Medical Review, 1998 Aug, 3:4.

40. Dr. Joseph Mercola, licensed Osteopathic physician and board-certified in family medicine, www.mercola.com.

41. Tim Griswold, former executive director of the Wisconsin Department of Commerce 'Dairy 2020 Initiative' commenting in the Wisconsin State Journal, USA, April 25, 2005.

42. Neal Barnard, M.D., Director of the Physician's Committee for Responsible Medicine. www.pcrm.org.

43. Amy Joy Lanou, Ph.D, Physicians Committee for Responsible Medicine, Dec. 2004.

44. Harvey and Marilyn Diamond, Fit For Life.

45. Julian Whiaker, M.D. Health & Healing, October, 1998, Volume 8, No. 10.

46. Acta Otolaryngol 1999: 119,8.

47. William Northrup, M.D., Natural Health, July 1994.

48. Gordon, The Case against Financing Dairy Projects in Developing Countries, 1999: a synthesizes of 428 peer-reviewed scientific papers concluding that milk drinking is a health hazard, 'even a threat of death' in later years, www.notmilk.com/wbstance.html.

49. Huijuan Xu, et al, American Journal of Epidemiology, Vol. 139, No.3 1994.

50. Dr. David Gordon, Milk and Mortality (ISBN 0-9671605-0-2 $35), Gordon Books (925-443-6213), 567 Amber Court, Livermore California 94550, USA.

51. There are many studies showing that dairy milk interferes with the production of oxytocin in the woman's body, and that oxytocin protects against breast cancer. Here are just a few of these studies: (1) Chow, S.Y. et al, Brain oxytocin receptor antagonism disinhibits sodium appetite in preweanling rats. Regul. Pept. 1997 / 68,119-124. (2) Arletti, R. et al, Influence of oxytocin on feeding behavior in the rat, Peptides 1989 / 10 (1) / 89-93. (3) Chua, S. et al, Influence of breastfeeding and nipple stimulation on postpartum uterine activity. Br. J. Obstet. Gynaecol. 1994 / 101 (9) / 804-805. (4) Moos, F.C. et al, Electrical recordings of magnocellular supraoptic and paraventricular neurons displaying both oxytocine- and vasopressin-related activity. Brain Res. 1995 / 669 (2) / 309-314. (5) Lindow, S.W. et al, Morphine suppresses the oxytocin response in breast-feeding women. Gynecol. Obstet. Invest. 1999 / 48 (1) / 33-37.

52. Winter, C K and S F Davis. 2006. Scientific status summary – Organic foods. J Food Sci 71(9):R117-R124.

53. Journal of Pediatrics, 1990, 116.

54. Acta Paediatrica, 1999 Dec, 88:12

55. Journal of Pediatric Surgery, 1999 Oct, 34:10

56. West Virginia Medical Journal, 1999 Sep-Oct; 95(5).

57. Townsend Medical Letter, May, 1995.

58. Frank Oski, M.D., Chief of Pediatrics at john Hopkins Medical School, *Don't Drink Your Milk*, July 1994.

59. Walene James, Immunization: the reality behind the myth, Bergin & Garvey, 1995, ISBN 0897893603.

60. Professor Carlo Leifert, et al, Newcastle University, UK, , March 2007, *Improving Sustainability in Organic and Low Input Food Production Systems*, part of the proceedings of the 3rd QLIF Congress, March 2007, University of Hohenheim, Germany.

61. The FSA (Food Standards Agency) is a UK government department responsible for providing advice and information on food safety 'from farm to fork'. The FSA works at 'arms length' from government because it doesn't report to a specific government minister, and is free to publish any advice it issues.

62. Milka M. Vidovic, et al, Heavy Metals in Relation to Soil – Fodder – Milk. Belgrade, Montenegro.

63. Heavy Metals in Soil by DIG-IT Magazine, PO Box 527, Augusta, NJ 07822, USA. www.dig-itmag.com

64. Polish Journal *Rocz Panstw Zakl Hig*, 1999, 50:3.

65. United Press International. March 11, 1983.

66. Steve Milloy, author of junkscience.com. Milloy tested samples of ice cream for dioxins and the results were reported in the Detroit Free Press, 11/8/99.

67. Journal of Animal Science, 1998 Jan, 76:1.

68. Hankinson. The Lancet, vol. 351. May 9, 1998.

69. Richard A. Scanlan, Ph.D. Dean of Research Emeritus and Professor of Food Science, *Nitrosamines & Cancer*, The Linus Pauling Institute.
70. Soil Association (UK), Organic Food & Farming, Myth vs Reality: the facts.
71. *The Milk Roadmap*, published by the 'Department for Environment, Food and Rural Affairs' UK, in September, 2007. Reported in The Times newspaper, 15 October 2007, p. 15.
72. Mulhall and Hansen, The Calcium Bomb, The Writers Collective, 2005, ISBN 1594111014.
73. [1] Gorner, F., Jencehova, J. and Nemeekova, K. (1977) "Changes in stored UHT milk", Prumysl Potravin 28(8), 441-445 (Fd. Science Abstr. 9 (3), p.414,1978). [2] Saeed Akhtar, et al, Physico-Chemical Changes In UHT Treated And Whole Milk Powder During Storage At Ambient Temperature, Journal of Research (Science), Bahauddin Zakariya University, Multan, Pakistan. Vol.14, No.1, June 2003, pp. 97-101 ISSN 1021-1012.
74. Robert O. Young Ph.D. and Shelley Redford Young, The pH Miracle, Time Warner 2002, ISBN 0751534064.
75. Feskanich D, et al, Milk, dietary calcium, and bone fractures in women: a 12-year prospective study, Am J Public Health. 1997 Jun;87(6):992-7.
76. [1] Rerkrai, S., Bassette, R. and Jeon, I.J. (1986) "Effects of various heat treatments in commercially processed UHT milk", J. Dairy Sci. 69 Suppl. (1), 63 (Dairy Sci. Abstr. 48 (11), p.6243, 1986). [2] Kocak, H.R. and Zadow, J.G. (1985) "Age gelatin of UHT whole milk as influenced by storage temperature", Australian J. Dairy Tech. 40, 14.

77. [1] Adhikari, A.K. and Singhal, O.P. (1992) "Effect of heat resistant microorganisms on the fatty acid profile and the organoleptic quality of UHT milk during storage", Indian J. Dairy Sci. 45(5), 272-277. [2] Gorner, F., Jencehova, J. and Nemeekova, K. (1977) "Changes in stored UHT milk", Prumysl Potravin 28(8), 441-445 (Fd. Science Abstr. 9 (3), p.414,1978).

78. Hofmekler, Ori, The Warrior Diet, Dragon Door Publications,U.S.; New Ed edition (30 Jan 2006), ISBN-13: 978-0938045489.

79. Solomon. Zaichkowsky, Polegato.Consumer Behavior: Pearson, Toronto. 2005. pg 39.

80. Belitz, Hand-Dieter, et al, Food Chemistry, p. 525, Springer 2004, ISBN 3540408185.

81. Chandan, Ramesh, Manufacturing Yogurt and Fermented Milks, p. 24, Blackwell Publishing, 2006, ISBN 0813823048.

82. *rBGH-Free Oregon Campaign*, Fact Sheet, Physicians For Social Responsibility, Oregon Chapter.

83. Belloque, J, et al, *Release of galactose and N-acetylglucosamine during the storage of UHT milk,* Instituto de Fermentaciones Industriales (C.S.I.C.), Spain,2001.

84. Da-Wen Sun, Thermal Food Processing: New Tehnologies And Quality Issues, CRC Press, 2006, ISBN 1574446282

85. Karl S Roth, MD, Professor, Department of Pediatrics, Creighton University School of Medicine, www.emedicine.com/ped/topic815.htm.

86. Neal Barnard, M.D., Director of the *Physician's Committee for Responsible Medicine.* www.pcrm.org.

87. Adhikari, A.K. and Singhal, O.P. (**1992**) "Effect of heat resistant microorganisms on the fatty acid profile and the organoleptic quality of UHT milk

during storage", Indian J. Dairy Sci. 45(5), 272-277. Ito, Y. (**1985**) "Studies on the keeping quality of UHT treated milk", Proceedings of the faculty of Agriculture, Kyushu Tokai University No.4, 111-116 (Dairy Science Abstr. 48(12), 1986).

88. Hofmekler, Ori, The Warrior Diet, Dragon Door Publications,U.S.; New Ed edition (30 Jan 2006), **ISBN-13:** 978-0938045489.

89. Morimoto, Richard, et al, Professor of Biology, Northwestern University, USA, *Molecular Mechanism Sheds Light On Neurodegenerative Diseases*, The EMBO Journal, a publication of the European Molecular Biology Organization, October 2004.

90. Rahman, Shafiur, CRC Press, 1999, ISBN 0824702093.

91. Lewis, M.J., Continuous Thermal Processing of Foods, Springer, 2000, ISBN 0834212595.

92. Caroli, Sergio, Element Speciation in Bioorganic Chemistry, Wiley, 1996, ISBN0471576417.

93. Buck, Albert Henry, A Treatise on Hygiene and Public Health, Ayer Publishing, 1977, ISBN 0405098103.

94. Kunz, Robert, *Protein: Reviewed by Neal Henderson MS CSC,* Alford Publishing, 2007, website:
http://www.snowshoemag.com/view_content.cfm ?content_id=311&printable=1

95. Nollen, Ellen A.A., et al, Genome-wide RNA interference screen identifies previously undescribed regulators of polyglutamine aggregation, Proc Natl Acad Sci U S A. 2004 Apr 27;101 (17):6403-8 15084750.

96. Bessie, B. Cook, et al, The Effect of Heat Treatment on the Nutritive Value of Milk Proteins,

Journal of Nutrition Vol. 44 No. 2 June 1951, pp. 217-235.

97. C. V, Morr, C.V., Functionality of Heated Milk Proteins in Dairy and Related Foods, Department of Food Science, Clemson University, Clemson, SC 29631, USA.

98. Richardson, T., Modification of whey proteins to improve functionality, 1984, Journal of Dairy Science, 67:2757-2774.

99. Chen, H, et al, Consumption of Dairy Products and Risk of Parkinson's Disease, American Journal of Epidemiology 2007 165(9):998-1006; doi:10.1093/aje/kwk089.

100. Mattila-Sandholm, T. & Saarela, M. (Eds.). (2003). *Functional Dairy Products.* New York: CRC Press.

101. O'Mahony, Frank, Milk Chemistry – An Introduction, ILCA Manual No. 4, ISBN 9290530928.

102. Saeed Akhtar, et al, PHYSICO-CHEMICAL CHANGES IN UHT TREATED AND WHOLE MILK POWDER DURING STORAGE AT AMBIENT TEMPERATURE, Journal of Research (Science), Bahauddin Zakariya University, Multan, Pakistan, Vol.14, No.1, June 2003, pp. 97-101 ISSN 1021-1012.

103. Dr. Patina Muhammad, N.D., C.Q.M (Certified Quantum Medicine), P.O. Box 65042, Phoenix, Arizona 85082-5042, USA.

104. Aiqian Ye, et al, Interactions of fat globule surface proteins during concentration of whole milk in a pilot-scale multiple-effect evaporator, Journal of Dairy Research (2004), 71: 471-479 Cambridge University Press.

105. Sung Je Lee, et al, *Chemical changes in bovine milk fat globule membrane caused by heat treatment and homogenization of whole*

milk, Journal of Dairy Research (2002), 69: 555-567 Cambridge University Press.

106.　　Fox, Patrick F. et al, Dairy Chemistry and Biochemsitry, Springer 1998, p. 349, ISBN 0412720000.

107.　　Fox, Patric F., *Fundamentals of Cheese Science*, Springer 2000, p.126, ISBN 0834212609.

108.　　Cano-Ruiz, M.E., et al, *Effect of Homogenization Pressure on the Milk Fat Globule Membrane Proteins*, Journal of Dairy Science Vol. 80, No. 11, 1997.

109.　　[1] Darling, D. F., et al, 1978, *Milk-fat globule membrane in homogenized cream*, J. Dairy Res. 45:197. [2] McPherson, et al,1984, *Isolation and composition of milk fat globule membrane material*, from Homogenized and Ultra Heat Treated Milks. J. Dairy Res. 51:289. [3] McPherson, A. V., et al,1983, *Reviews of the progress of dairy science; the bovine milk fat globulemembrane – its formation, composition, structure, and behaviour in milk and dairy products*. J. Dairy Res. 50:107. [4] Sharma, R., H., et al, 1996, *Composition and structure of fat globule surface layers in recombined milk,* J. Food Sci. 61:28. [5] Sharma, S. K., et al, 1993, *Interactions between milk serum proteins and synthetic fat globule membrane during heating of homogenized whole milk*, J. Agric. Food Chem. 41:1407.

110.　　Gorski, Donna, *Food scientists: don't forget about homogenization - milk processing,* Dairy Foods, August, 1994.

111.　　Doctoral Dissertations, Mitchell Memorial Library, Mississippi State University, USA, 1980

112.   Spreer, Edgar, Milk and Dairy Product Technology, CRC Press, 1998, ISBN 0824700945.

113.   Goodall, Chris, *How to Live a Low-Carbon Life: The Individuals Guide to Stopping Climate Change*, 2007, ASIN: B000WXMZDK.

114.   [1] Hammarlun, Ray, A Study of Marketing Issues with Organic Milk, Dept. of Agricultural Economics, Kansas State University, AGMRC 2002. [2] Glaser and Thompson, Demand and Conventional Beverage Milk, Selected Paper presented at Western Agricultural Association annual meeting, Vancouver, Canada, 2000.

115.   Avery, Alex, Director of Research and Education, Hudson Institute, *Nature's Toxic Tools: The Organic Myth of Pesticide-Free Farming*, Center for Global Food Issues, P.O. Box 202, Churchville, Va 24421-0202, USA.

116.   Robertson, Gordon L., *Food Packaging: Principles and Practice*, CRC Press, 2006, ISBN 0849337755.

117.   Dairy Processing Handbook, published by Tetra Pak Processing Systems AB, S-221 86 Lund, Sweden.

118.   [1] Datta, Nivedita, Deeth, Hilton, C. et al, Australian Journal of Dairy Technology. Vol. 57: No 3. (October 2002), *Ultra-high-temperature (UHT) treatment of milk: comparison of direct and indirect modes of heating.* [2] Williams, R.P.W., Australian Journal of Dairy Technology, Vol. 57: No. 1 (April 2002), *The relationship between the composition of milk and the properties of bulk milk properties.* [3] Datta, Nivedita, Deeth, Hilton, C., Food and Bioproducts Processing: Transactions of the Institution of Chemical Engineers, Vol. 79: Part C, *Age Gelation of UHT Milk: A Review.* [4]]Fry, M.R., Institute of Food

Technologists Annual Meeting, 1995, *Relaunching an old product and awakening consumer interest in improved technology: the Parmalat experience.* [5] *Journal of Agriculture and Food Chemistry,* Vol 52, pages 3702-3070, 2004.

119.   García-Risco, Mónica R, et al, *Proteolysis, protein distribution and stability of UHT milk during storage at room temperature,* Instituto de Fermentaciones Industriales (CSIC), Juan de la Cierva 3, E-28006 Madrid, Spain.

120.   Singh, R, et al, *Kinetics of lipid hydrolysis during storage of UHT milk,* Journal of Food Science and Technology (Mysore), 2004 (Vol. 41) (No. 2) 139-142.

121.   Belloque, J, et al, *Release of galactose and N-acetylglucosamine during the storage of UHT milk,* Instituto de Fermentaciones Industriales (C.S.I.C.), Juan de la Cierva 3, 28006 Madrid, Spain, Oct. 2000.

122.   Particle for use as a milk fat globule substitute, composition containing same and process for the preparation of said particle, United States Patent 5534501, http://www.freepatentsonline.com/5534501.html

123.   Fox, P.F., *Fat Globules in Milk,* Elsevier Science, 2002.

124.   McGee, Harold, On Food and Cooking: The Science and Lore of the Kitchen, Scribner, 2004, ISBN 0684800012.

125.   Nauta, W.J. et al, *Consequences Of Converting To Organic Dairy Farming For Production, Somatic Cell Count And Fertility Of First Parity Holstein Cows,* 2005, Louis Bolk Institute, Department of Animal Husbandry, Hoofdstraat 24, NL-3972 LA Driebergen, The Netherlands.

126.   Dr. Michael Greger,M.D., general practitioner specializing in clinical nutrition and a founding member of the American College of Lifestyle Medicine. Website: http://www.drgreger.org.

127.   [1] Rozzi, Paola, Ph.D. *A Selection Index for Organic Dairy Farms in Ontario.* [2] Hardeng F. and V.L. Edge, 2001, *Mastitis, chetosis and milk fever in 31 organic and 93 conventional Norwegian dairy herds,* J. Dairy Sci. 84: 2673-2679.

128.   Gastroenterology.

129.   [1] Deeth, H.C., *Homogenized Milk and Atherosclerotic Disease: A Review,* Otto Madsen Dairy Research Laboratory *Department* of Primary Industries Hamilton, Queensland, 4007 Australia. [2] Oster, K. A. 1971. *Plasmalogen diseases: A new concept of the etiology of the atherosclerotic process,* Am. J. Clin. Res. 2:30.

130.   Dr. John H. Maher (DCCN, Vice President, Education, BioPharma Scientific, Inc, www.biopharmasci.com) email to the author Russell Eaton dated 27 December 2007.

131.   Thompson, A.K. et al, *Preparation of Liposomes from Milk Fat Globule Membrane Phospholipids Using a Microfluidizer,* J. Dairy Sci. 89:410–419, American Dairy Science Association, 2006.

132.   Professor Douglas Goff, Dairy Science and Technology Education, University of Guelph, Canada, www.foodsci.uoguelph.ca/dairyedu/home.html.

133.   Global Food Markets, Leatherhead Food International, Surrey, United Kingdom, www.globalfoodmarkets.com.

134.   Kristensen, T. and Struck Pedersen, S., *Organic dairy cow feeding with emphasis on*

Danish conditions, The 4th NAHWOA Workshop, Wageningen, Denmark, 24-27 March, 2001.

135. Foulkes, E.C., *Transport of Toxic Heavy Metals Across Cell Membranes*, Department of Environmental Health, College of Medicine, University of Cincinnati, Cincinnati, Ohio 45267–0056, USA

136. [1] Souza V, Bucio L, Gutierrez-Ruiz MC, Cadmium uptake by a human hepatic cell line, Toxicology 120:215–220, 1997. [2] Blazka ME, Shaikh ZA. Differences in cadmium and mercury uptakes by hepatocytes: Role of calcium channels. Toxicol Appl Pharmacol 110:355–363, 1991.

137. Marie-Caroline Michalski and Caroline Janue, *Science et Technologie du Lait et de l'Œuf*, Agrocampus Rennes, Trends in Food Science & Technology, Volume 17, Issue 8, August 2006, Pages 423-437.

138. Hillman, Howard, *The new kitchen science*, P. 104, Houghton Mifflin Books, 2003, ISBN 061824963X.

139. Hunter, J. 0, Food allergy - or enterometabolic disorder? The Lancet 1991; 338: 495-96.

140. Dr. Ethan D. Feldman,D.C., *Regaining Balance: Natural Approaches to Treating Female Athlete Triad Syndrome in Dancers*,www.dcdoctor.com/dc/ca/backnaction_com/rightpages/dancemed_regainingbalance.html.

141. Sandra, S., Dalgleish, D. G., *Effects of ultra-high-pressure homogenization and heating on structural properties of **casein** micelles in reconstituted skim milk powder.* International Dairy Journal, 2005 (Vol. 15) (No. 11) 1095-1104.

142. Email to the author from the UK Dairy Council dated 10 January 2007 explaining how casein is deigested.

143.   Natural Health School (An Online Course in Herbalism, Nutrition & Natural Health) www.naturalhealthschool.com.

144.   Cavallo, M.G., et al, *Cell-mediated immune response to beta casein in recent-onset insulin-dependent diabetes: implications for disease pathogenesisk,* 1996, The *Lancet.* 348 (9032) 926-8.

145.   Butler, Dr. Justine, *White Lies,* 2006, published by the Vegetarian & Vegan Foundation, Top Suite, 8 York Court,Wilder Street, Bristol BS2 8QH, UK.

146.   Wahle, K.W., Heys, S.D. and Rotondo, D. 2004, *Conjugated linoleic acids: are they beneficial or detrimental to health?* Progress in Lipid Research, 43 (6) 553-87.

147.   [1] Shargel, Leon, et al, Comprehensive Pharmacy Review, Lippincot Williams & Wilkins, 2006, ISBN 0781765617. [2] Ulf Risérus, MMed, et al, 2002, *Supplementation With Conjugated Linoleic Acid Causes Isomer-Dependent Oxidative Stress and Elevated C-Reactive Protein,* American Heart Association Journals, 01.CIR.0000033589.15413.48v1. [3] A *natural quick fix - What Doctors Don't Tell You,* HealthWorld Online.

148.   Mougios V, Matsakas A, Petridou A, et al. *Effect of supplementation with conjugated linoleic acid on human serum lipids and body fat.* J Nutr Biochem 2001;12:585–94.

149.   Quignard-Boulange, Annie, et al, *Les isomères conjugués de l'acide linoléique (CLA).* Conférence, INCONNU (11/2004) 2005, vol. 12, n°1, pp. 45-50 [6 page(s) (article)] (ref. 40).

150.   Market Scope Europe Ltd., ISSN 1366-5634, editor: Brian R. Hicks, Website: www.crop-protection-monthly.co.uk.

151.   Michalski,   Marie-Caroline,   et   al,   Does homogenization   affect   the   human   health properties of cow's milk?   Trends in Food Science & Technology, Volume 17, Issue 8, August 2006, Pages 423-437.

152.   Michalski, Marie-Caroline, On the supposed influence of milk homogenization on the risk of CVD, diabetes and allergy, British Journal of Nutrition (2007), 97: 598-610.

153.   ByeDr.com,   *Medicine   Questions   and Answers*,   website: www.byedr.com/Diet-Fitness/119-diet.html.

154.   Martin, S., *Intestinal Permeability*, BioMed Newsletter Issue No. 11, May 1995.

155.   Ellis, Kathryn A, et al, *Investigation of the vitamins A and E and β-carotene content in milk from UK organic and conventional dairy farms*, University of Glasgow study: Journal of Dairy Research (2007), 74:484-491, CUP.

156.   Research carried out by the *Danish Institute of Agricultural Research*, 2005, Soil Association annual   conference,   held   by   University   of Newcastle's Quality Low Impact Food (QLIF) Congress in Newcastle. Project leader: was Prof. Carlo Leifert, QLIF project leader.

157.   Johnson L (1991) "Thermal degradation of carotenes and influence on their physiological functions." *Adv Exp Med Biol,* vol. 289, pp. 75-82.

158.   K. A. Ellis, K.A. et al, *Comparing the Fatty Acid Composition of Organic and Conventional Milk*, J. Dairy Sci. 89:1938–1950, American Dairy Science Association, 2006.

159.   Benbrook, Charles, *Simplifying the Pesticide Risk Equation: The Organic Option*, Foreword by Dr Alan Greene, The Organic Center, USA, March 2008. This is a 49 page report that can be downloaded by going to www.organic-center.org.

160. Butler, Gillian, et al, Newcastle University, *Fatty acid and fat soluble antioxidant concentrations in milk from high and low input conventional and organic systems; seasonal variation*, J. of the Science of Food and Agric., manuscript ID JSFA-07-0595.R2, April, 2008.

161. [1] Roche, JR, et al, *'High input farming - the road to a better life: more money, more options'*, Proceedings of the South Island Dairy Event, Invercargill, New Zealand, Pp 120-131, June, 2002. [2] Cederberg, C., *Life cycle assessment of milk production - a comparison of conventional and organic farming.* Report by the Swedish Institute for Food and Biotechnology, 1998, SIK, Gothenburg, Sweden.

162. Open letter to the milk industry and to the U.S. Ohio State Milk Review Committee in particular. The letter, titled *"Milk: Let the buyer (the environment, the cow) beware"* was released around 2 April, 2008. It was signed by sixty-six university dairy and veterinary scientists from just about every major land grant university in the USA plus over 65 additional academic scientists in animal science and veterinary medicine who urge consumers to make informed science-based decisions when purchasing milk. The letter was coordinated by dairy medicine Prof. John Fetrow of the University of Minnesota and Dairy and Animal Science Department Head Terry D. Etherton of Penn State University, and signed by leading academics including Dale Bauman of Cornell University in New York, one of the pioneers in studying cow hormones in milk.

163. Burger, Liza, *A longer life for dairy*, article published in M&J Retail, USA, November, 2007.